CHILDHOOD CHAMPIONS

VEGETARIAN COOKBOOK

GEORGE GREEN & CHEF JEFFRIE TONEY

Published by Echo Books.

Echo Books is an imprint of Superscript Publishing Pty Ltd, ABN 76 644 812 395

Registered Office: Registered Office: PO Box 669, Woodend, Victoria, 3442.

www.echobooks.com.au

Creator: George Green and Jeffrie Toney, authors.

Title: Childhood Champions : Vegetarian Cookbook.

ISBN: 978-1-922603-18-0 (paperback)

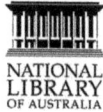

A catalogue record for this book is available from the National Library of Australia

Layout and design by Peter Gamble, Canberra.
Set in Garamond Premier Pro Display

Created by: George Green. Written by: George Green.
Co-writer: Jeffrie Toney.
www.echobooks.com.au

www.littleglobalpeople.com
Instagram: @littleglobalpeople

www.cheftoneycatering.com

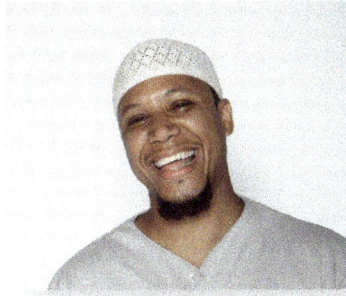

George Green is an **African-American author and motivational** speaker from New York City. He is the Co-founder of Little Global People, unique books and entertainment where kids of color are represented.

George not only inspires through his words but also through his dedication in giving back to the community. George holds a bachelor's degree in English and Psychology from Auburn University.

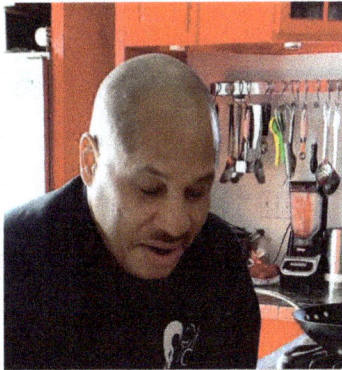

Jeffrie Toney, a distinguished, **African American** chef hailing from Detroit, Michigan, has carved out a culinary niche by mastering the art of French cuisine. As the visionary behind Chef Toney's Catering and beacon of inspiration, he not only tantalizes taste buds with his delectable creations but also enriches his local community through philanthropic endeavors. A proud holder of a bachelor's degree in culinary arts from the Culinary Institute of America, Chef Toney's influence extends far beyond the kitchen.

Bismillah

In the name of Allah, the most gracious, most merciful all praise is for Allah, Lord of the worlds, the most gracious the most merciful. All glory is to Allah (SWT).

The *Childhood Champions Vegetarian Cookbook* is dedicated to my daughter Aminaah and Chef Jeffrie Toney's children Justin, Saskia and Empress.

I'd like to thank my wife Mei Nee for her unlimited support, and Chef Jeffrie Toney.

Contents

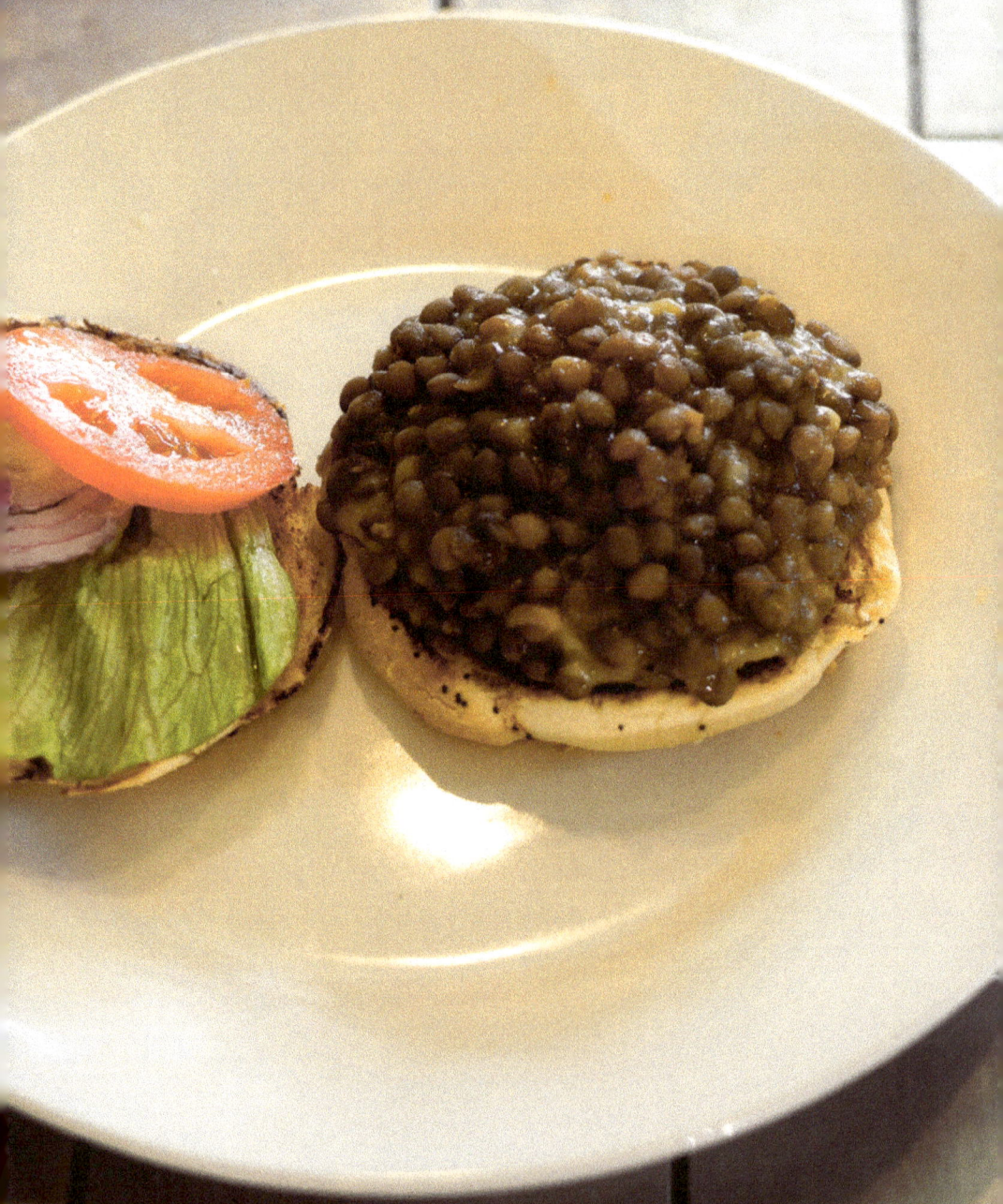

Vegetarian Lentil Sloppy Joe

Prepping Time: 10 minutes

Ingredients:

- 1 cup lentils

Directions:

- Precook lentils
- Add BBQ sauce or your favorite sauce
- Toast hamburger bun
- Assemble

Cooking Time: 6-8 minutes

Serves: 1 Person

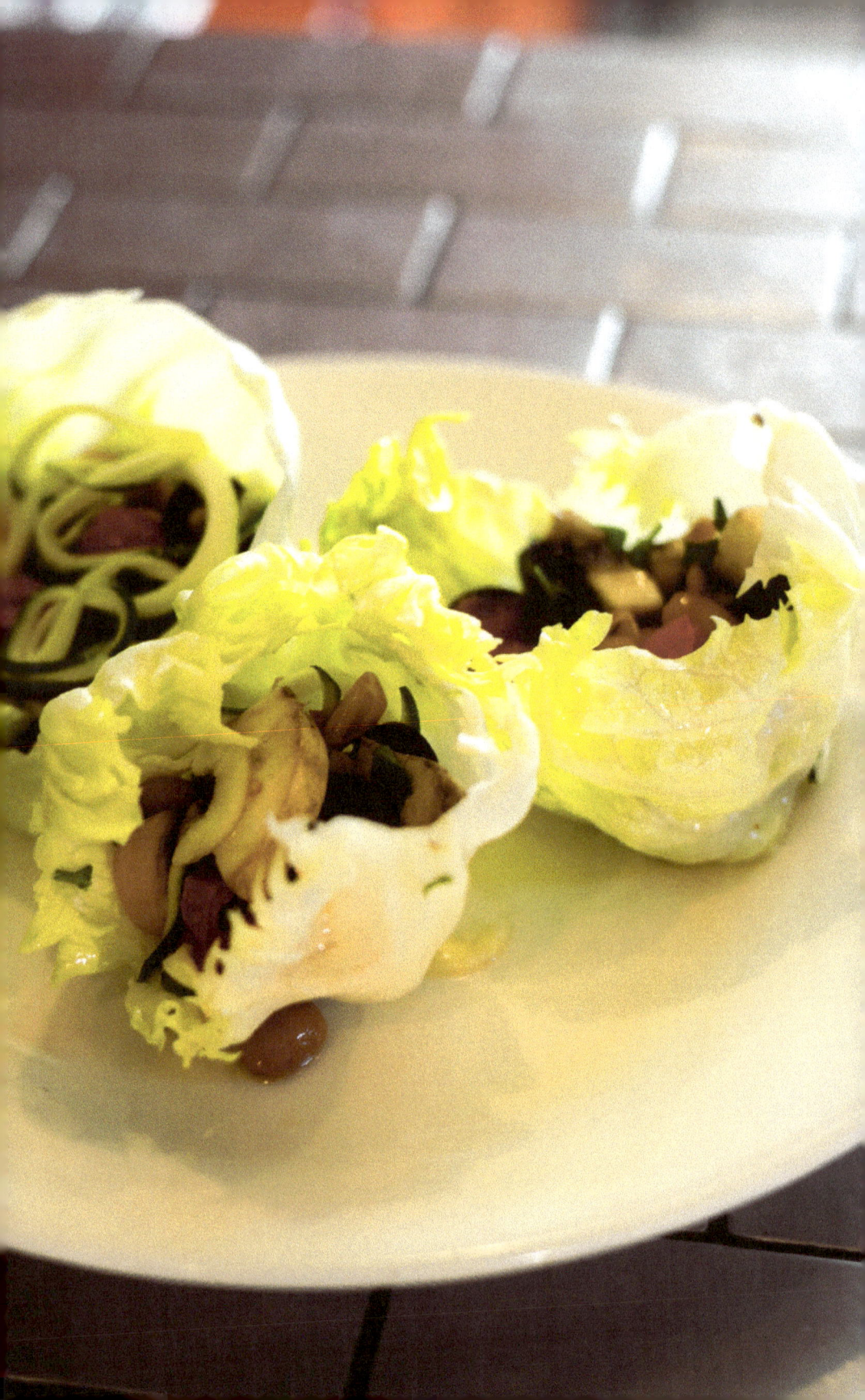

Vegetarian San Choy Bow

Prepping Time: 10 minutes

Ingredients:

- ½ Cup of beans
- ½ Cup of black olives
- ½ Cup of mushrooms
- ½ Cup of diced tomatoes
- 1 Head of lettuce (cut out the center to create a bowl)

Directions:

- Mix all ingredients in a bowl
- Add favorite dressing
- Place mixture into lettuce bowl

Cooking Time: 10 minutes

Serves: 2 people

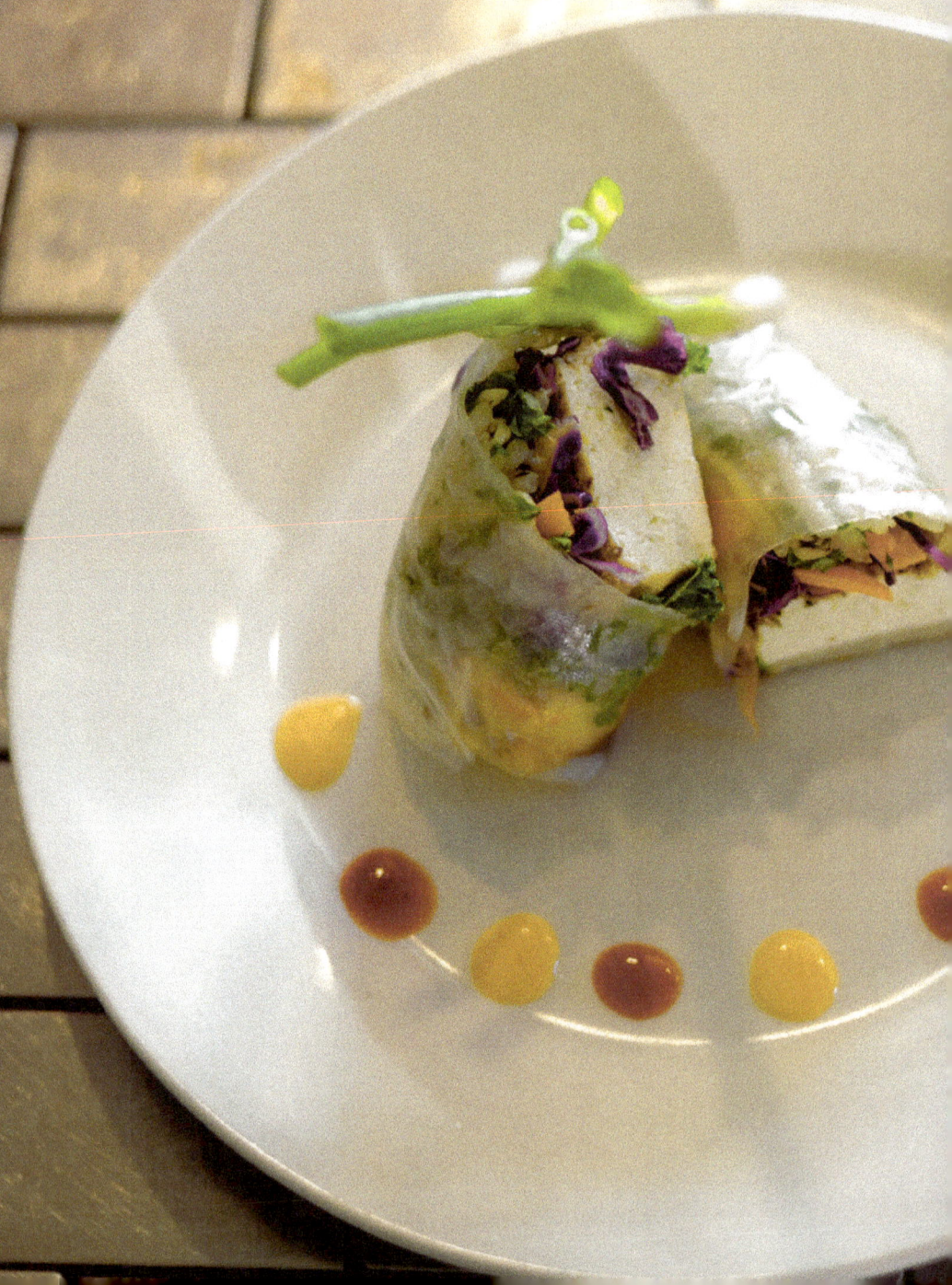

Stuffed Tofu & Vegetable Rice Paper Wraps

Prepping Time: 20 minutes

Ingredients:

- Desired vegetables
- Tofu
- Olive oil (2 tablespoons)
- Salt & pepper (for taste)

Directions:

- Drain & slice tofu into desired size
- Mix tofu & desired vegetables in a bowl
- Add tofu & vegetable mix in rice paper
- In a hot pan with olive oil, sear off wrap until brown on all sides
- Sprinkle with salt & pepper (for desired taste)

Cooking Time: 10 minutes

Serves: 2 people

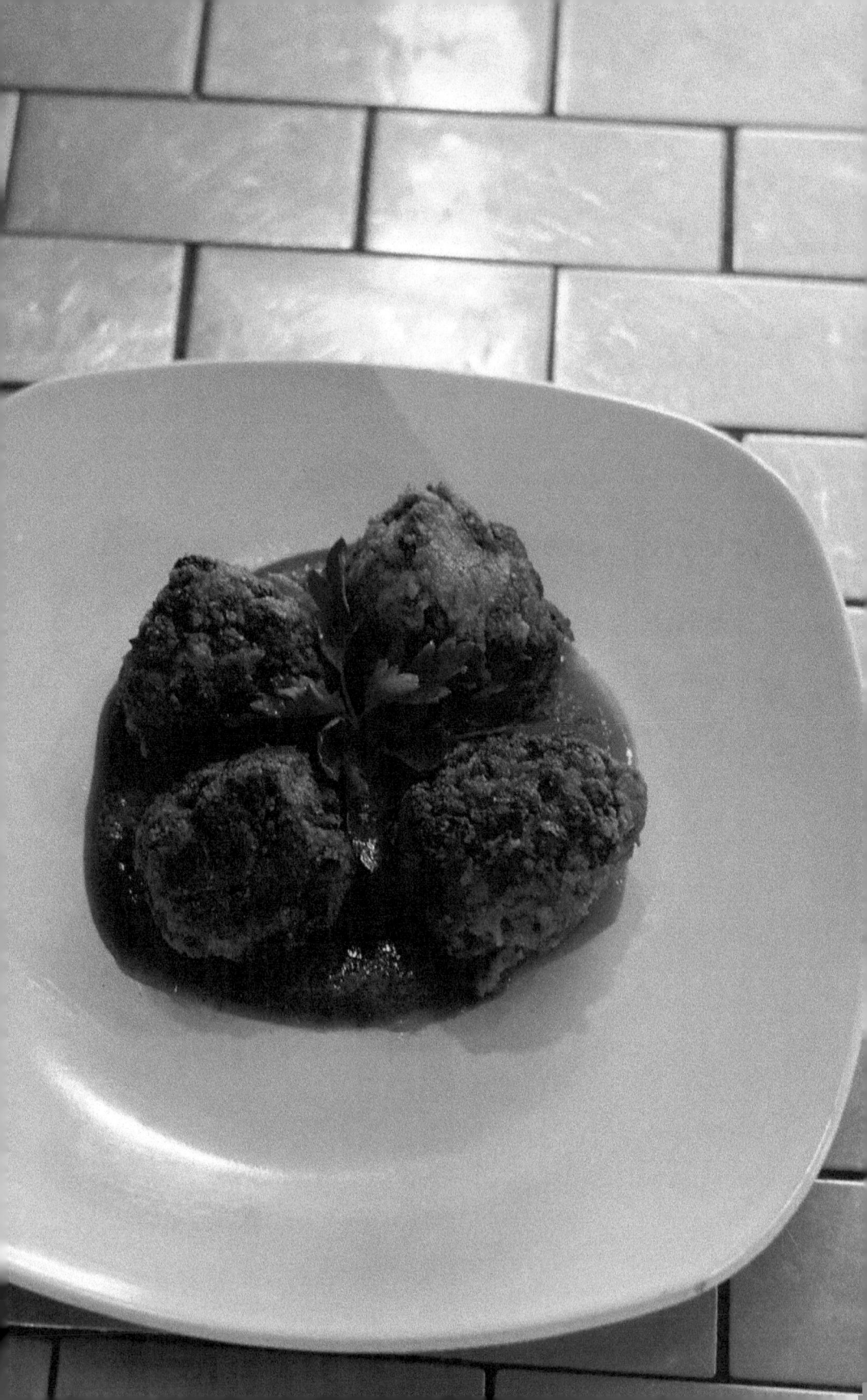

Vegetarian Meatballs

Prepping Time: 20 minutes

Ingredients:

- 1 Cup of roasted sweet potatoes (peeled)
- 1 Cup of black beans
- Cooking oil
- Flour of choice
- Salt & pepper (for taste)

Directions:

- In a mixing bowl add all ingredients for meatballs and use your hands to mix well
- Use hands to roll the mixture into meatballs of equal sizes
- Lightly flour
- Heat oil in a pan and sear the meatball under medium heat
- Sprinkle with salt & pepper (for desired taste)

Cooking Time: 10 minutes

Serves: 2 People

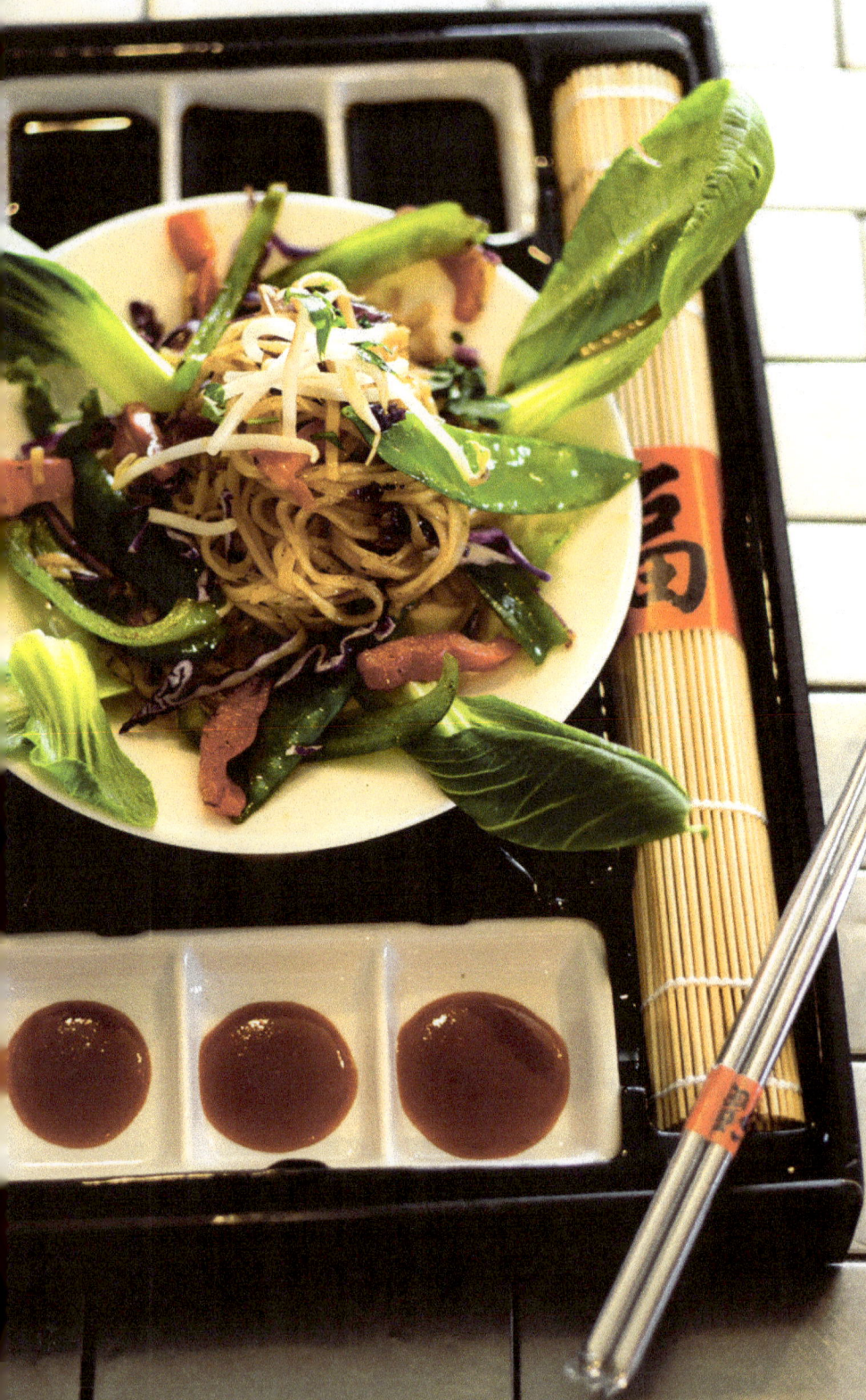

Vegetarian Chow Mein Stir-fry

Prepping Time: 20 minutes

Ingredients:

- ½ Green bell pepper (Capsicum)
- ½ Red bell pepper (Capsicum)
- ½ White or yellow onion
- 1 Small red cabbage
- 1 Bok Choy
- 1 Clove of minced garlic
- 1 ½ Bean sprouts
- Soy sauce
- 2 tablespoons of vegetable oil
- Chow Mein noodles

Directions:

- Prepare the noodles: Bring a large Wok or pot of water to a boil
- Cook noodles for 1 minute, transfer to a strainer (colander)
- Rinse the cooked noodles with cold water until totally cool
- Transfer to a large sheet tray
- Drizzle with 1 tablespoon of oil to prevent sticking and toss to coat
- Slice vegetables into 1/2 inch thick strips
- Add a remaining 1-tablespoon of oil to the hot Wok. Add vegetables & stir-fry for 30-seconds
- Add the cooked, drained noodles to the Wok and toss to combine stirring until the noodles are toasty and totally dry, about 2 minutes
- Add soy sauce
- Sprinkle with salt & pepper (for desired taste)

Cooking Time: 15 minutes

Serves: 2 people

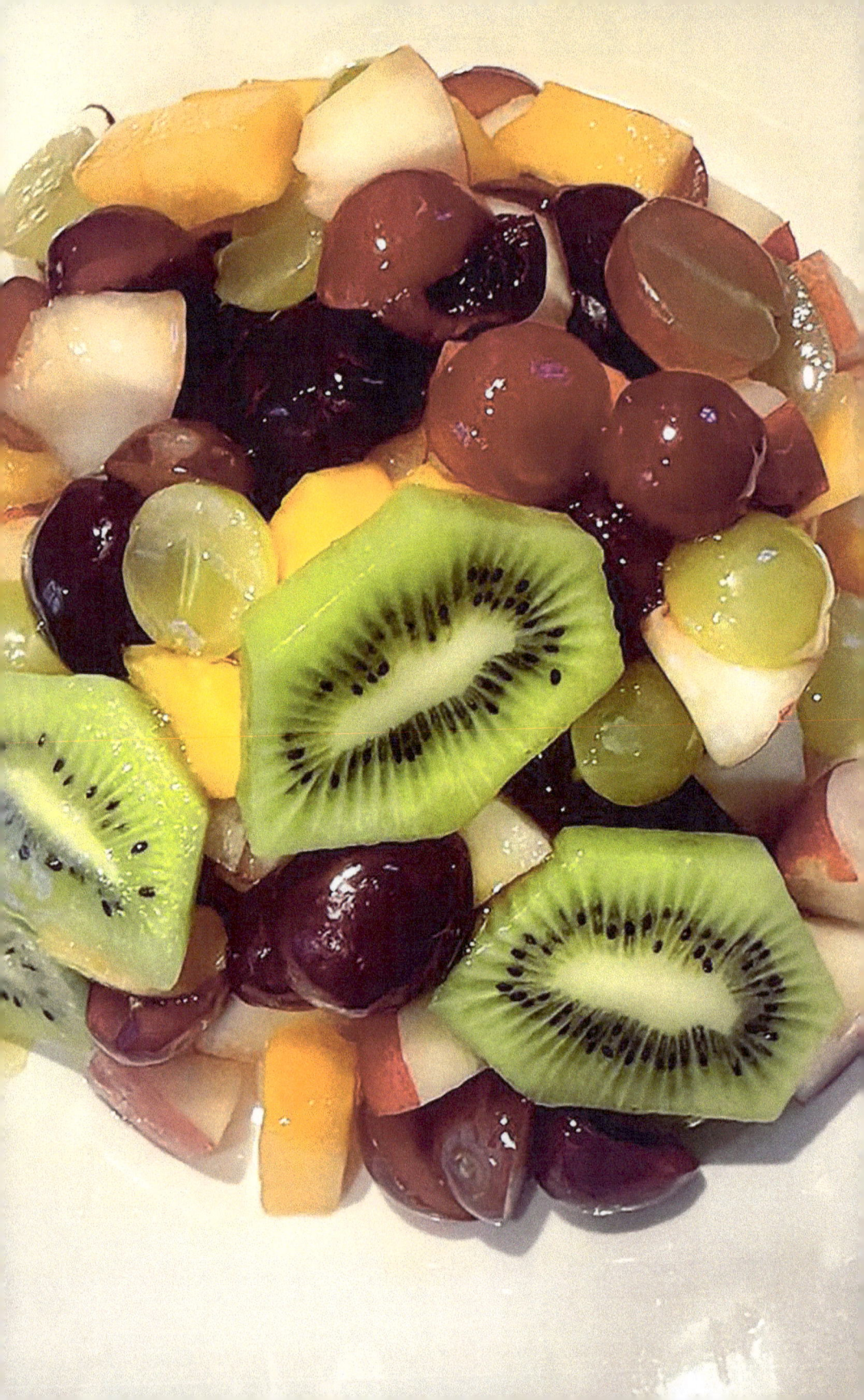

Fruit & Honey Salad

Prepping Time: 4-5 minutes

Ingredients:

- 1 Cup of green grapes
- 1 Cup of red grapes
- ½ Cup of chopped cantaloupe or (rock melon)
- ½ Cup of deseeded cherries
- 2 Peeled & chopped kiwi
- 1 Squeezed lemon
- Drizzle raw honey to taste and mix

Directions:

- Rinse all fruit
- Dry the fruit
- Cut fruit and toss with honey

Serves: 2-4 People

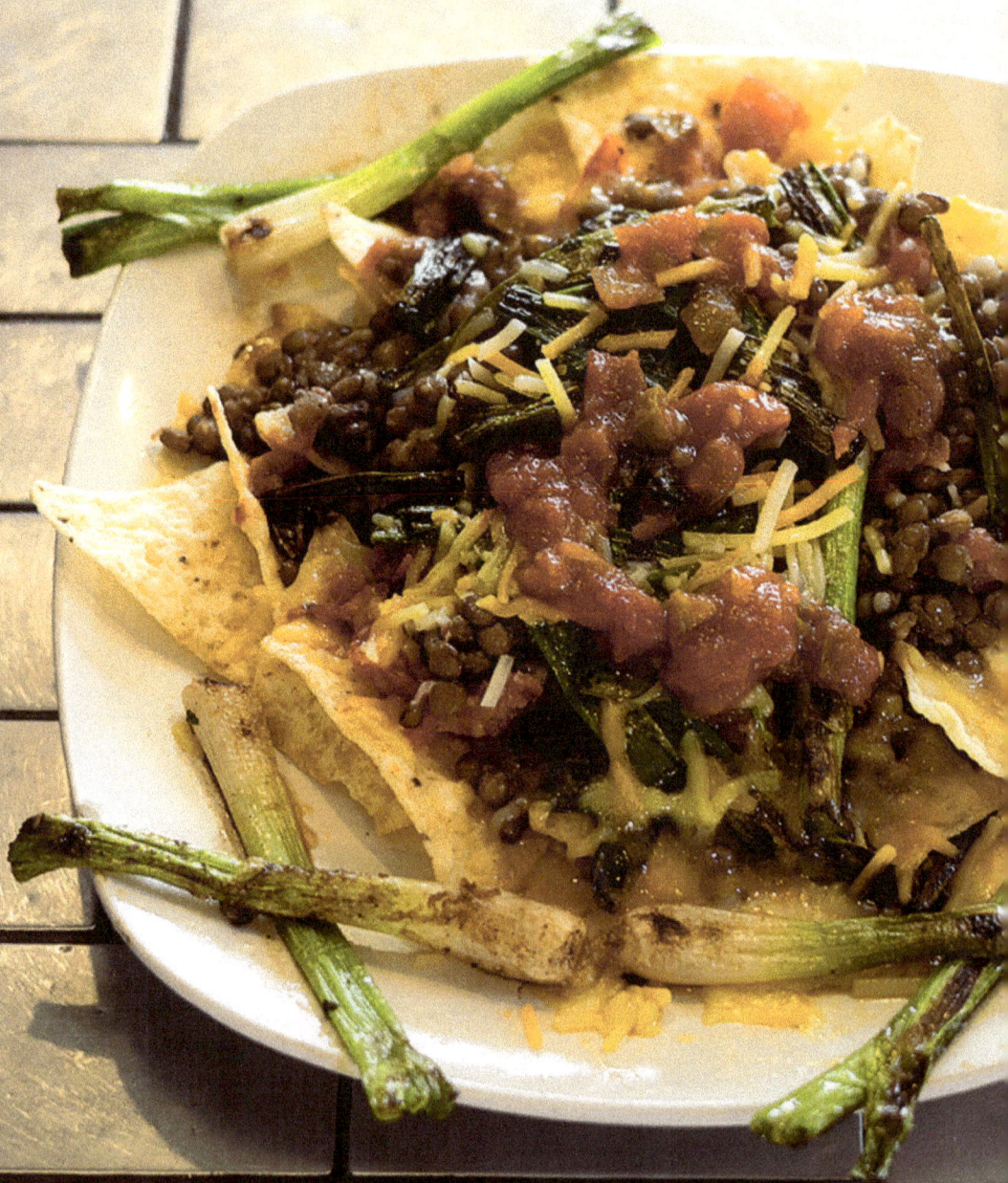

Vegetarian Lentil Nachos

Prepping Time: 20 minutes

Ingredients:

- ½ Cup of diced tomatoes
- 1 Cup of lentils
- ½ Bag of green onions chopped
- ½ Cup of plant based cheese
- ½ Bag of corn chips
- Taco sauce

Directions:

- Pre-cook lentils
- In a mixing bowl, add tomatoes, lentils & green onions & mix well
- Place corn chips on a plate
- Add toppings and sprinkle cheese on top
- Drizzle with taco sauce

Cooking Time: 8 minutes

Serves: 2 people

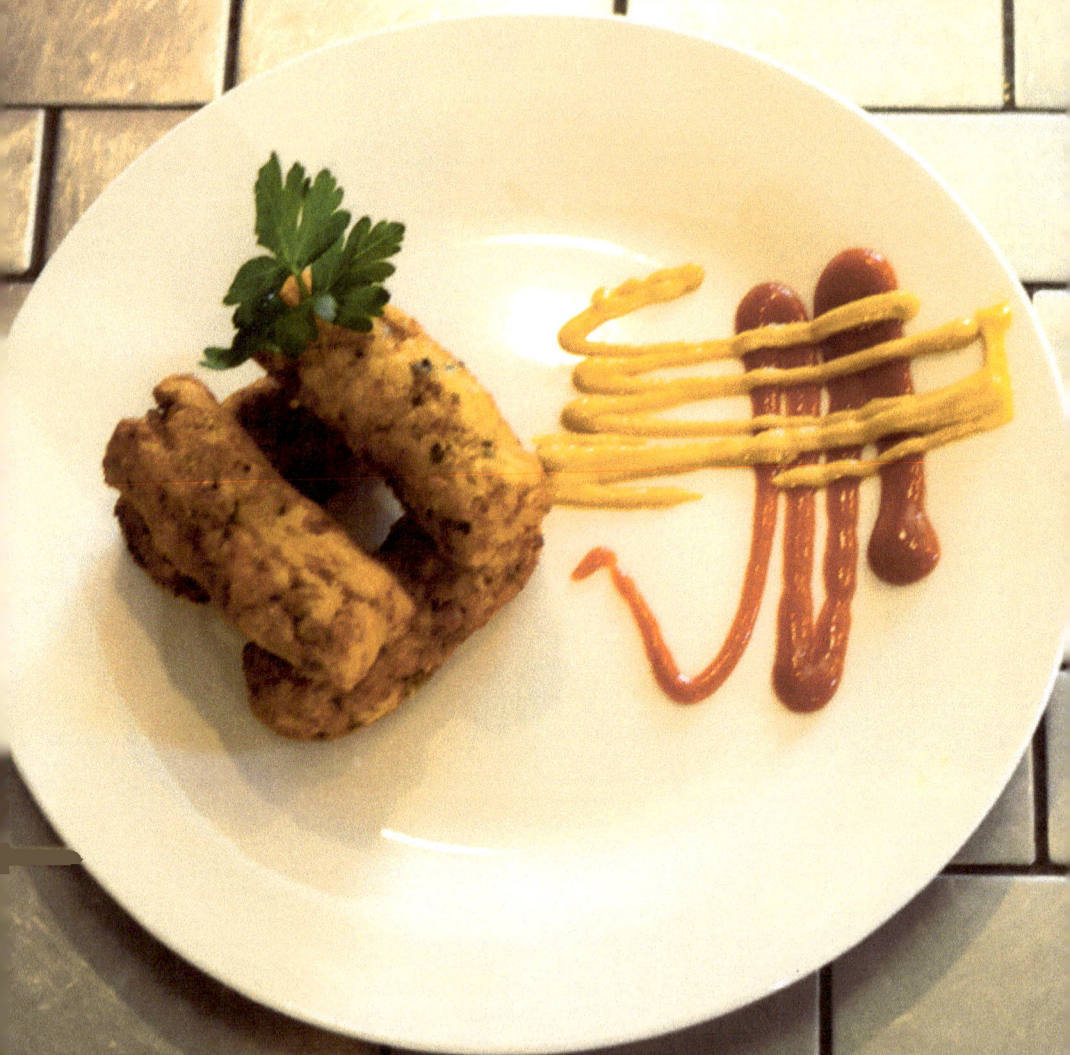

Vegetarian Nuggets

Prepping Time: 15 minutes

Ingredients:

- ½ Cup of sweet potato (precooked)
- ½ Cup of brown rice (precooked)
- ¼ Cup of black-eyed peas
- ½ Cup of chick pea flour
- 1 Egg
- ½ Cup of bread crumbs

Directions:

- Preheat oven to 400 degrees (F) or (204 degrees Celsius) line a baking sheet with parchment paper
- Scoop about 1 tablespoon of the sweet potato mixture and shape into a nugget
- Bake the nuggets for 20 minutes, flipping halfway until golden brown
- Let the nuggets cool for 5 minutes before serving with your choice of dipping sauce

Cooking Time: 20 minutes

Serves: 2 people

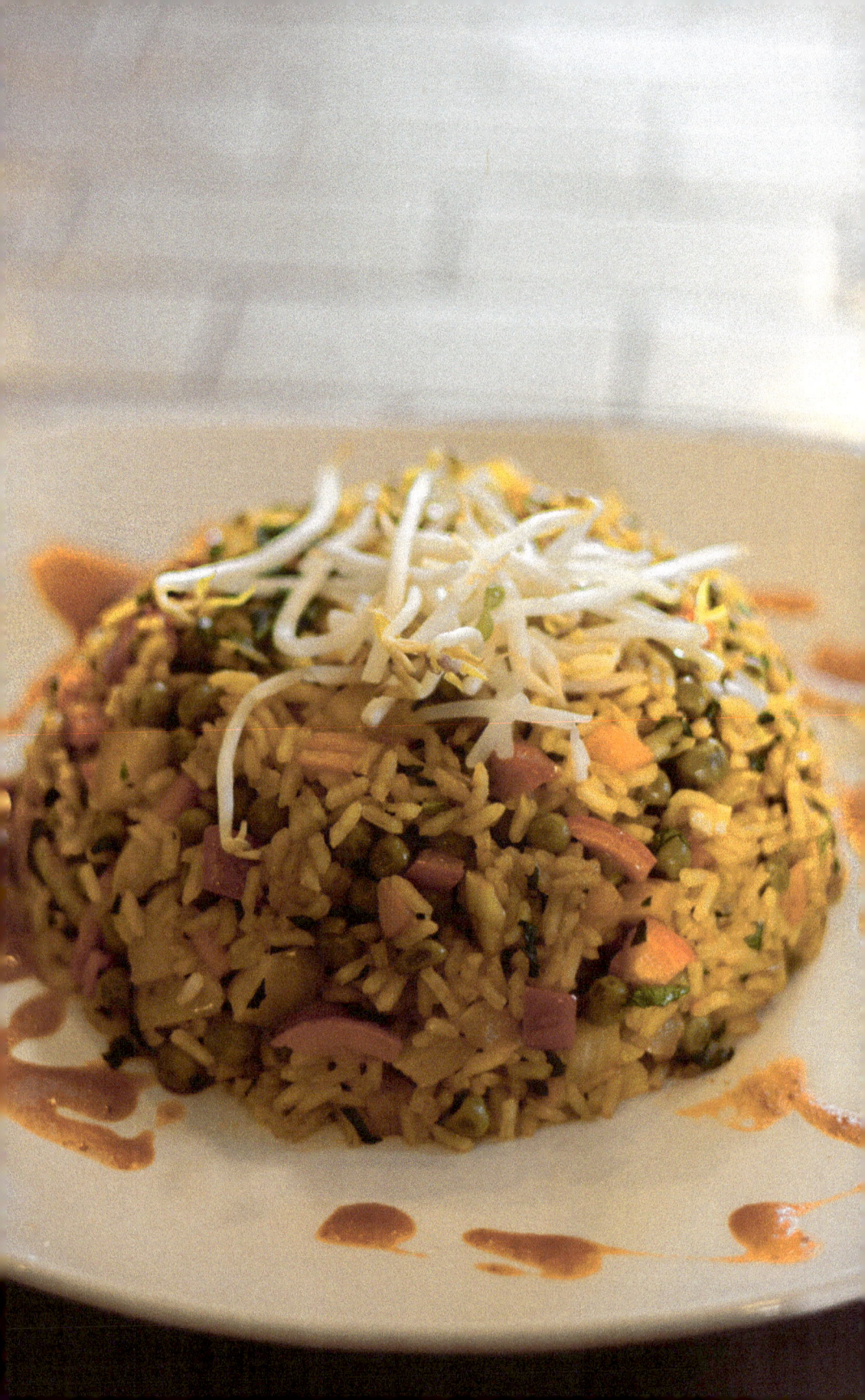

Vegetarian Fried Rice

Prepping Time: 10 minutes

Ingredients:

- 2 Teaspoons of olive oil
- ½ Cup of diced carrots
- ½ Cup of diced yellow onion
- 1 Tablespoon of minced garlic
- ½ Cup of diced bell pepper
- ½ Cup of snow peas
- 3 Cups of cooked rice
- 2 tablespoons of soy sauce
- Black pepper (for taste)

Directions:

- Use a Wok or deep skillet to heat the oil over high heat until shimmering
- Add carrots, onions and garlic while cooking until the onion is glassy looking
- Add the bell peppers (capsicum) and vegetables while cooking for 3-4 minutes until tender
- Add the peas, rice, soy sauce, black pepper and mix well
- Let the rice cook until slightly crispy

Cooking Time: 8 minutes

Serves: 4 people

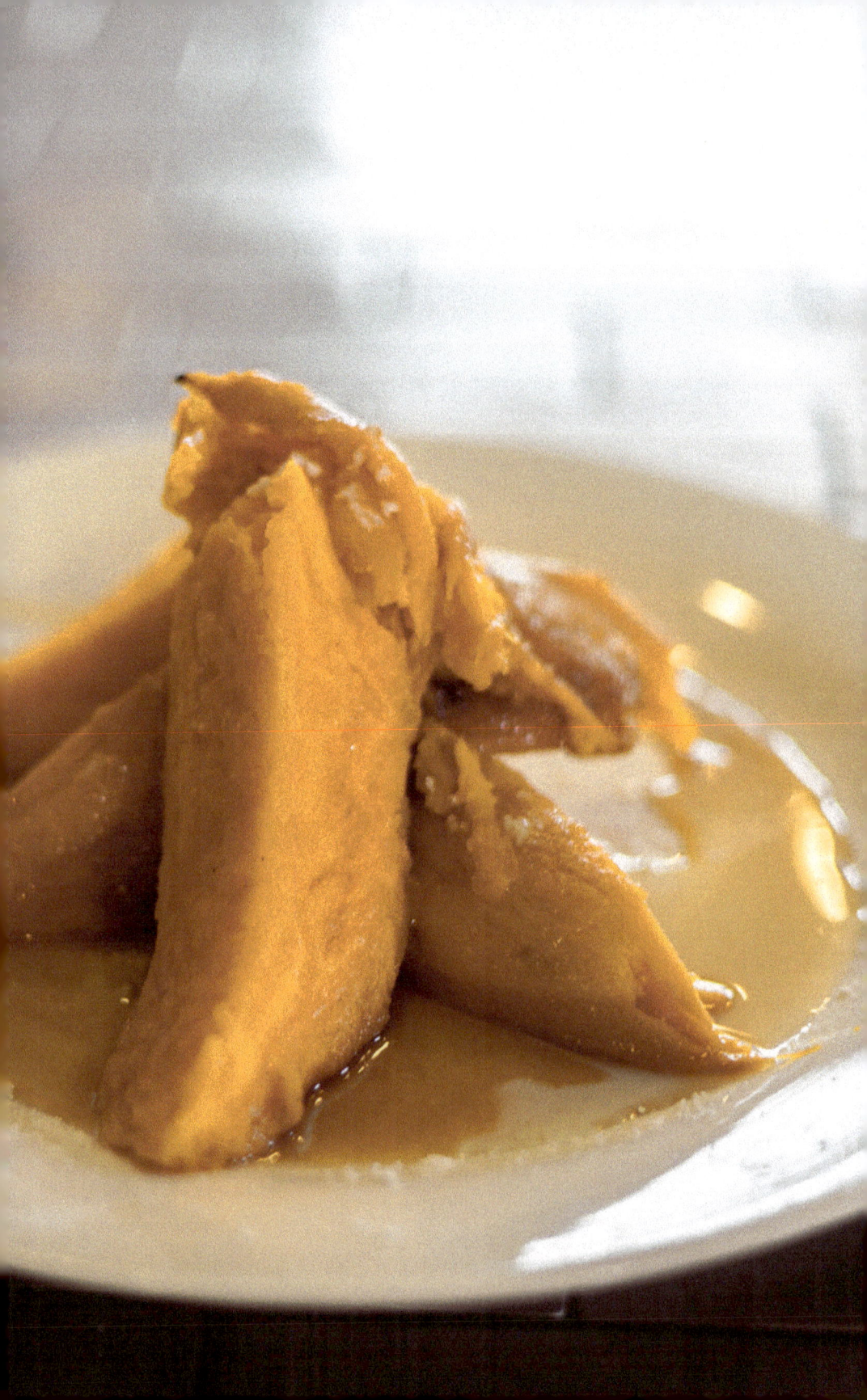

Honey Glazed Sweet Potatoes

Prepping Time: 5 minutes

Ingredients:

- 2 Large, sweet potatoes
- 1 Tablespoon of brown sugar
- 1 Tablespoon of butter
- 4 Tablespoon of honey

Directions:

- Preheat over to 350 degrees (F) or (176 degrees Celsius) Line a baking sheet with parchment paper
- Baked sweet potatoes in oven for 45 minutes or until tender
- Remove and let cool for 10 minutes
- Peel and slice sweet potatoes (about 1-inch thick)
- Melt butter and pour over sweet potatoes
- Dust sweet potatoes with brown sugar
- Drizzle with honey

Cooking Time: 45 minutes

Serves: 4 people

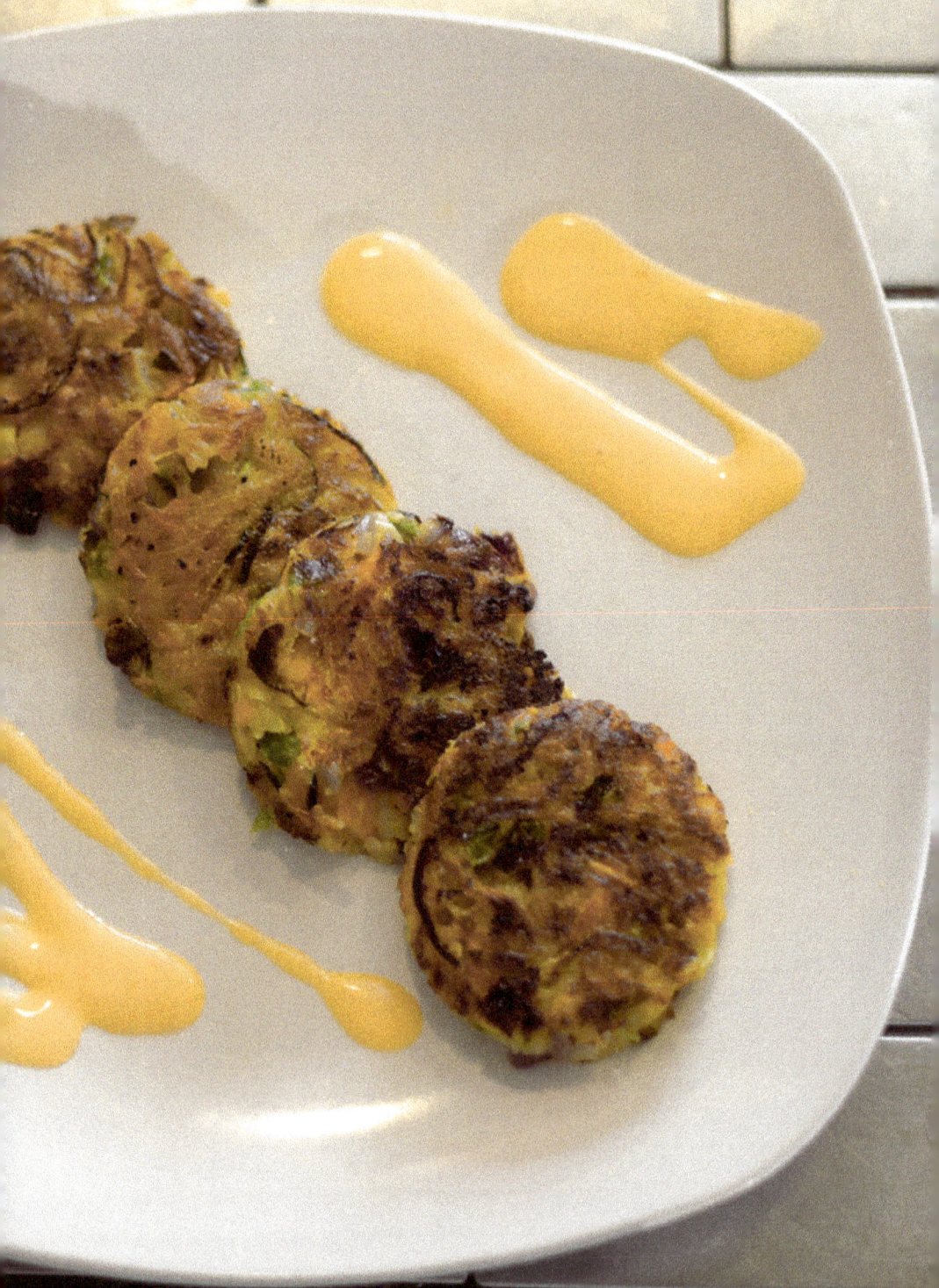

Vegetarian Fritters

Prepping Time: 20 minutes

Ingredients:

- 2 Cups of shredded zucchini
- 1 Cup of shredded carrots
- 1 Cup of shredded potatoes
- ¼ Cup of onions
- ¼ of bell peppers (capsicum)
- 2 tablespoons of chickpea flour
- ⅓ Cup of almond milk
- Salt & pepper (for taste)
- ½ tablespoon of cumin
- 2 large eggs, lightly beaten
- 2 tablespoons of vegetable oil or more as needed

Directions:

- Combine vegetable, chickpea flour and eggs in a bowl until well mixed and season with salt, pepper and cumin
- Heat 2 tablespoons of vegetable oil in a large non stick pan over medium heat
- Drop 3 tablespoons full of the zucchini batter into a non stick pan flattening each dollop with the back of a spoon
- Pan-sear until golden brown for 1 to 2 minutes per side
- Transfer fritters to a paper towel lined plate to drain and cool slightly before serving

Cooking Time: 10 minutes

Serves: 4 people

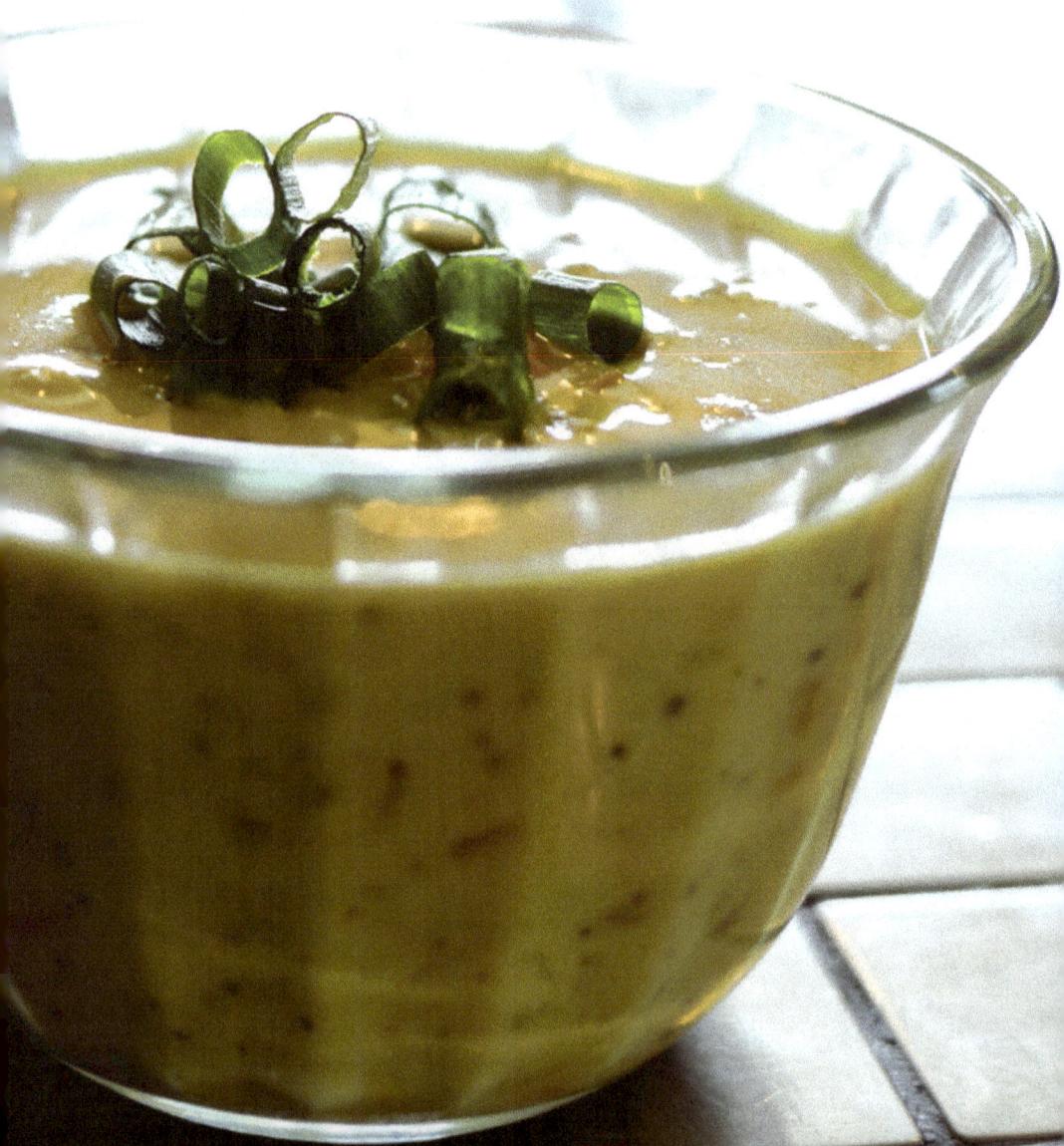

Coconut Curry Soup

Prepping Time: 10 minutes

Ingredients:

- 3 Tablespoons of butter
- ½ Medium onion roughly chopped
- ¾ Pound of carrots, peeled and cut into ½ inch circles and ¼ cup of onions
- 1 Tablespoon of minced garlic

- 2 Cups of vegetable stock
- 1 Cup of unsweetened coconut milk and add salt & pepper (for taste)
- 1 Teaspoon of peeled grated fresh ginger
- Salt & pepper (for taste)

Directions:

- Heat the butter until the foam subsides. Add the diced chopped onions, sprinkle with salt, and stir the mixture
- Add the chopped carrots along with the spices. Stir and cook until softened about 10 minutes
- Add the stock. There should be enough broth to cover the vegetables
- Bring the pot to a boil over high heat. Reduce the heat to medium and continue cooking until the carrots until tender about 5 to 10 minutes
- Wait until the soup cools slightly and puree in a food processor or blender
- Add enough coconut milk and a little more stock if necessary to to add consistency
- Adjust seasoning to desired taste

Cooking Time: 20 minutes

Serves: 2 People

23

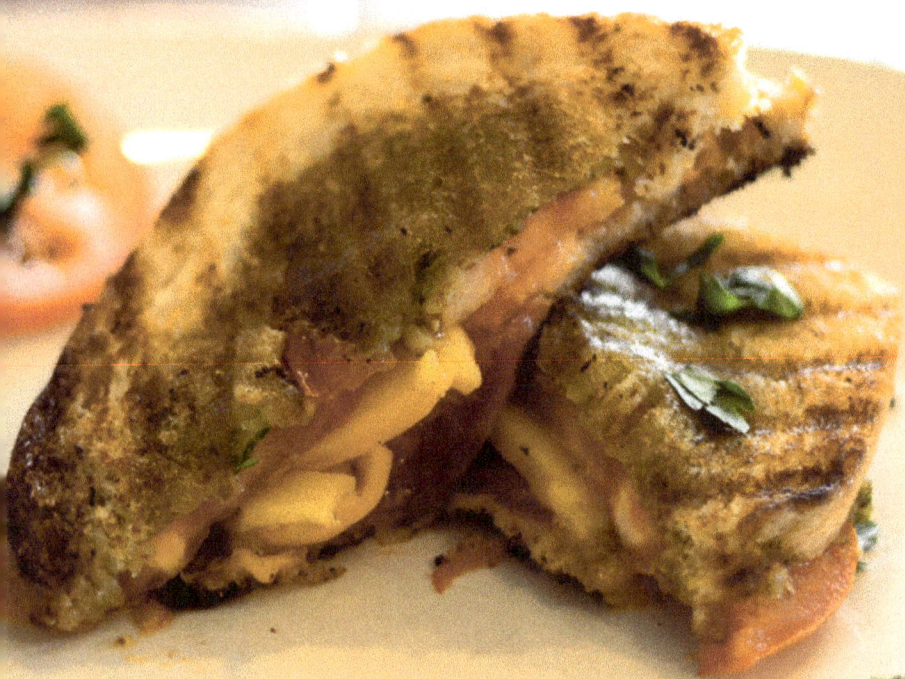

Tomato Basil
Grilled Cheese Sandwich

Prepping Time: 10 minutes

Ingredients:

- 2 Slices of bread
- 2 Slices of tomato
- 2 Slices of plant-based cheddar & smoked gouda cheese
- 2 Leaves of fresh chopped basil
- 1 ½ Tablespoon of butter
- 1 Tablespoon of Pesto
- Salt & pepper (for taste)

Directions:

- On 2 slices of bread, spread pesto & layer cheese and tomatoes, sprinkle with basil, salt and pepper
- In a skillet over medium heat, melt butter & toast sandwich until golden brown on both sides and cheese is melted

Cooking Time: 10 minutes

Serves: 1 person

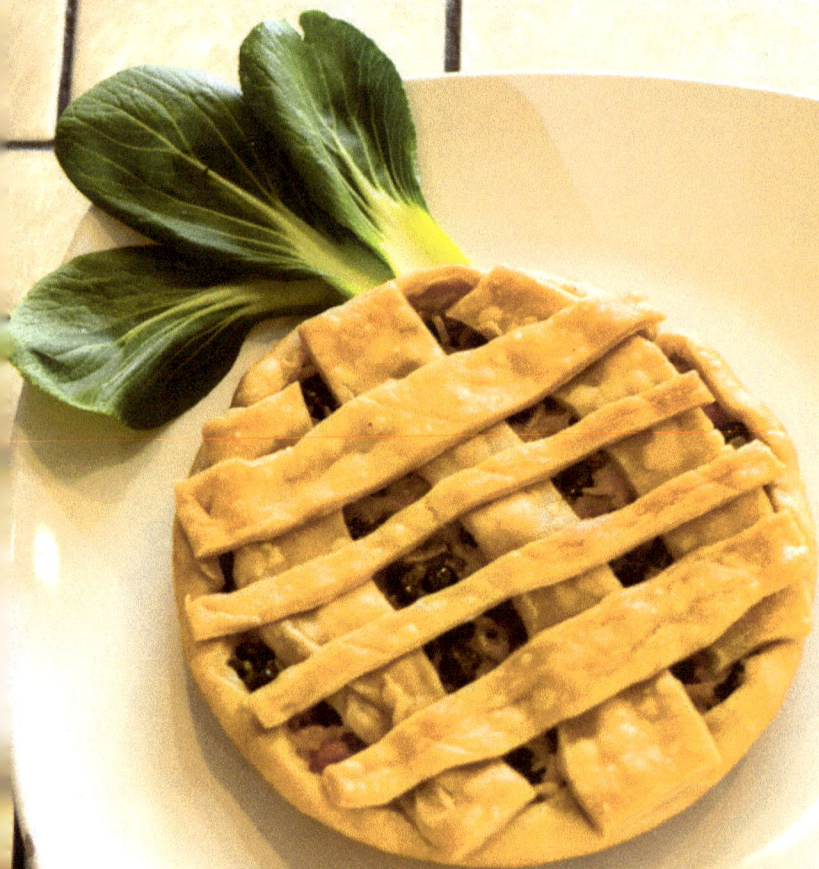

Lentil Curried Pie

Prepping Time: 30 minutes

Ingredients:

- 1 Cup of brown rice precooked
- 1 Cup of precooked lentils
- 1 Cup of carrots
- 1 Cup of peas
- 1 Tablespoon of coconut oil
- ½ Tablespoon of curry

- ½ Cup of minced onion
- ½ Tablespoon of minced garlic
- ½ Cup of coconut milk
- 1 Pie crust
- ½ Cup of chickpea flour
- Salt & pepper (for taste)

Directions:

- Preheat over to 350 degrees (F) or (176 degrees Celsius)
- Heat oil in a large pan, then cook the onion and garlic over medium heat
- Add carrots & ½ pt of water, bring to a boil then simmer for 5 minutes until the vegetables are almost tender
- Drain, reserving the cooking liquid, then mix with the peas
- Melt butter in a small pan, stir in flour, then cook for 1 minute. Add reserved vegetables cooking liquid, then cook and stir until if forms a thick sauce. Season with salt, pepper & curry. Remove from heat and then cool
- Add all ingredients to a mixing bowl and mix well
- Spoon the mixture into a pie crust and cover with remaining dough and press firmly to seal. Make a hole in the center of the pie to allow steam to escape
- Brush with butter, place on a baking sheet and bake for 30-40 minutes

Cooking Time: 40 minutes

Serves: 4 People

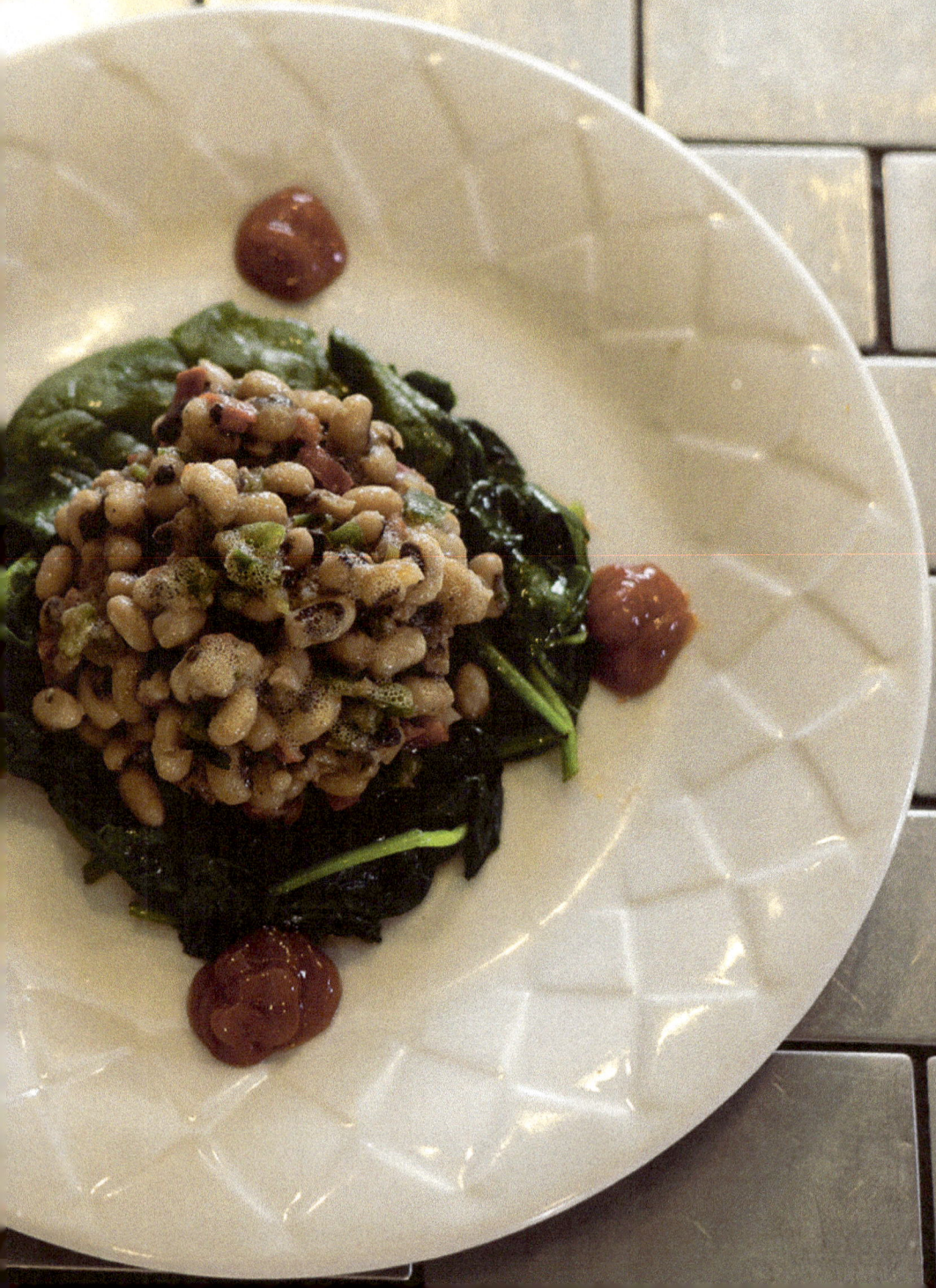

Black Eyed Pea Salad

Prepping Time: 2 Hours

Ingredients:

- 2 Cups of black-eyed peas
- 2 Tablespoons of chopped green onions
- 1 Small red & green bell pepper (capsicum) finely chopped
- 1 Tablespoon of minced garlic
- 1 Tablespoon of olive oil
- Salt & pepper for taste

Directions:

- Place black-eyed peas in a large bowl and add 3 cups of water for every cup of peas. Cover and place in the refrigerator, and let the beans soak for 1 hour
- Once your beans are done soaking, rinse and drain them. Add them to a pot over the stove and cover with at least two inches of water
- Simmer until the beans are tender for about 1 hour
- Add all ingredients to a mixing bowl with olive oil
- Toss all together with the black-eyed peas and let them marinate in the refrigerator before serving
- Season with salt & pepper (for taste)

Cooking Time: 1 Hour

Serves: 4 People

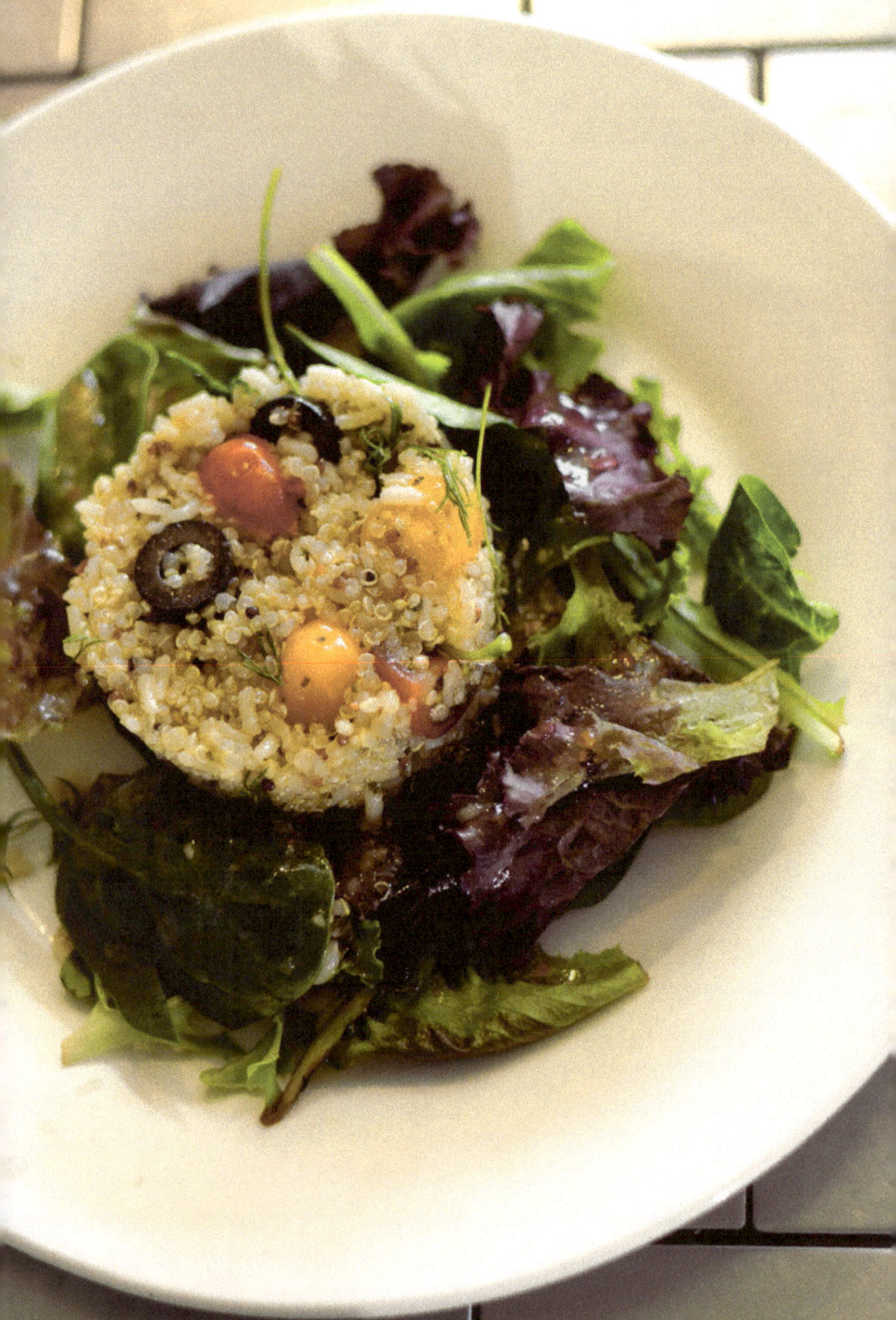

Quinoa Salad

Prepping Time: 10 minutes

Ingredients:

- 2 Cups of cooked quinoa
- 2 Cups of fresh salad greens
- 1 Cup of cherry tomatoes (halves)
- 1 Cup of chopped cucumber
- 1 Cup of chopped red onion
- Add salt & pepper (for taste)
- Add Light salad dressing

Directions:

- Use a large salad bowl and combine quinoa, salad greens, cucumber, tomatoes and red onions
- Drizzle salad with light dressing and gently toss until salad is coated with the dressing
- Season with salt & pepper (for taste) then serve

Cooking Time: 10 minutes

Serves: 6 People

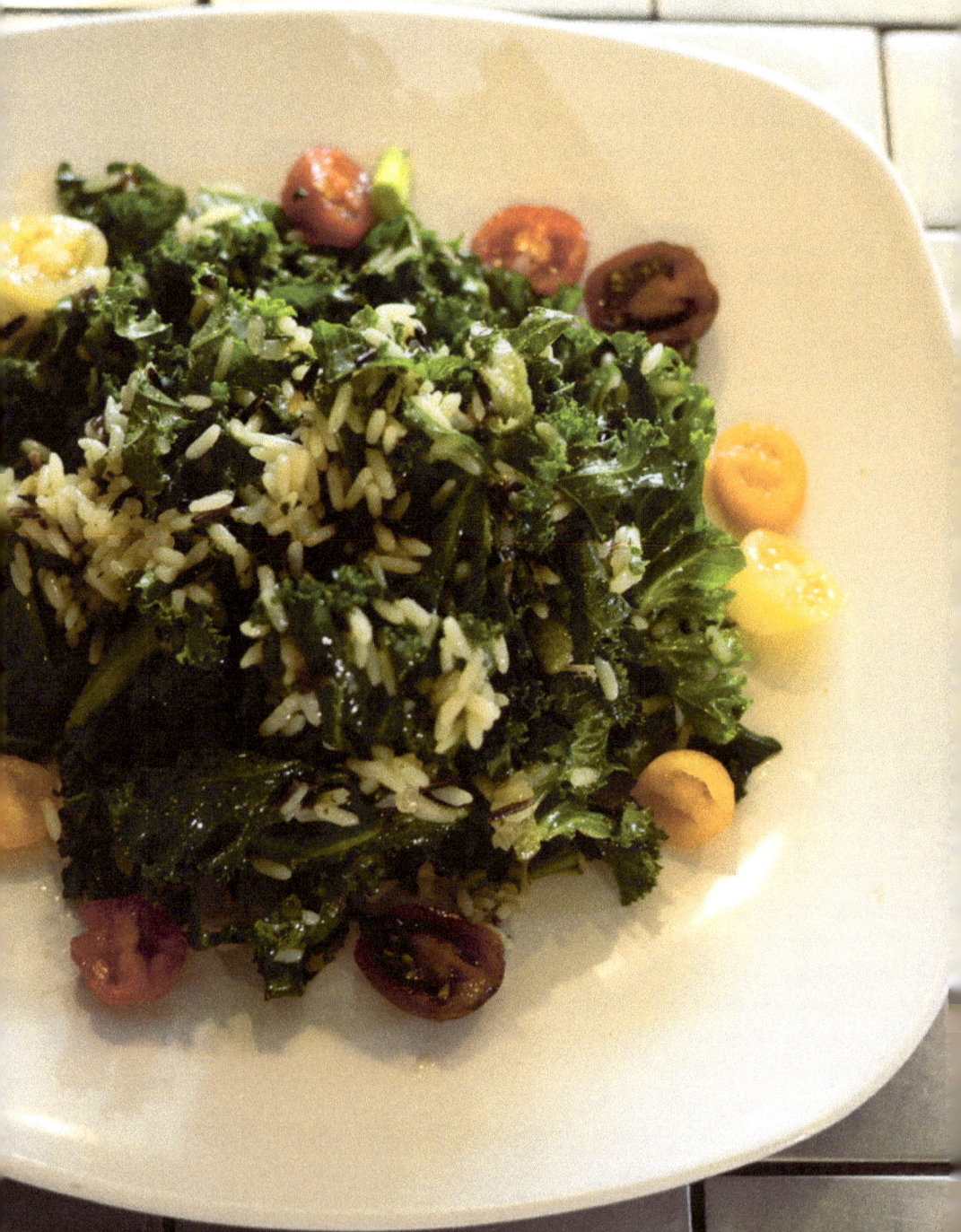

Wild Rice and Kale Salad

Prepping Time: 10 minutes

Ingredients:

- ½ Cup of cooked wild rice
- 2 Cups of Kale
- 2 Tablespoons of roasted red pepper (capsicum)
- Add salt & pepper (for taste)

Directions:

- Cook the rice according to the instructions & let cool
- Add the kale to a bowl and drizzle dressing while adding a pinch of salt
- Toss the kale until it becomes tender
- Add the wild rice to the remaining dressing & mix well
- Season with salt & pepper to desired taste and serve

Cooking Time: 15 minutes

Serves: 3 People

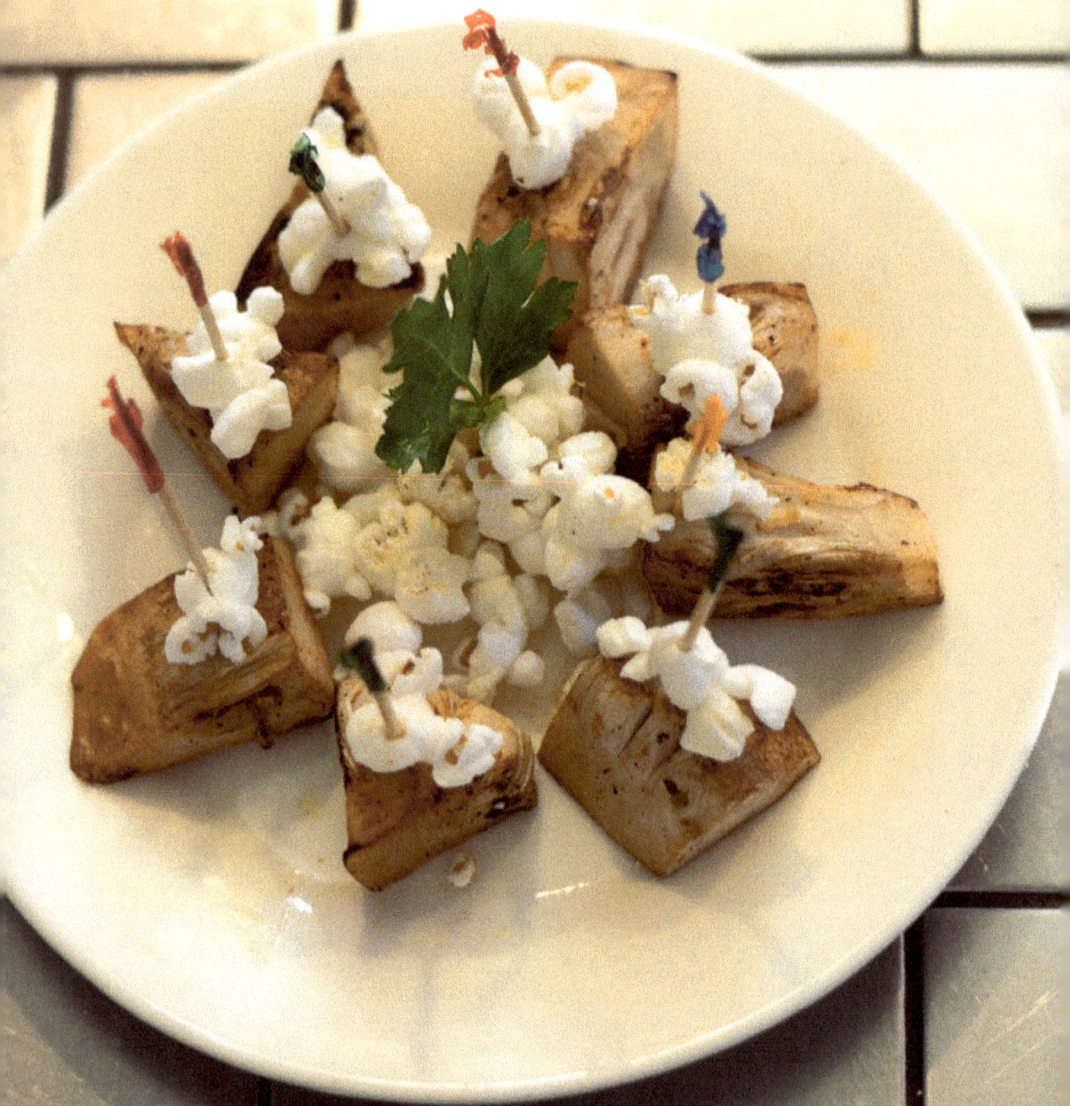

Jack Fruit Popcorn Bites

Prepping Time: 15 minutes

Ingredients:

- 2 Cups of young jack fruit
- 1 Bag of popcorn
- ¼ Teaspoon of salt
- ½ Teaspoon of onion powder
- ½ Teaspoon of garlic powder
- ½ Tablespoon of vegan chicken powder
- 2 Tablespoon of chickpea flour

The batter

- ¼ Cup of chickpea flour
- ½ Teaspoon of dried oregano
- 2 Tablespoon of cornstarch
- A pinch of salt & pepper

Directions:

- Whisk the batter ingredients in a bowl until smooth consistency
- Heat about 1 inch of oil or more in a shallow frying pan until hot
- Place Jack fruit pieces into batter and then hot oil
- Cook for about 1 minute on each side until crispy then transfer to paper towel

Cooking Time: 3 minutes

Serves: 3-4 People

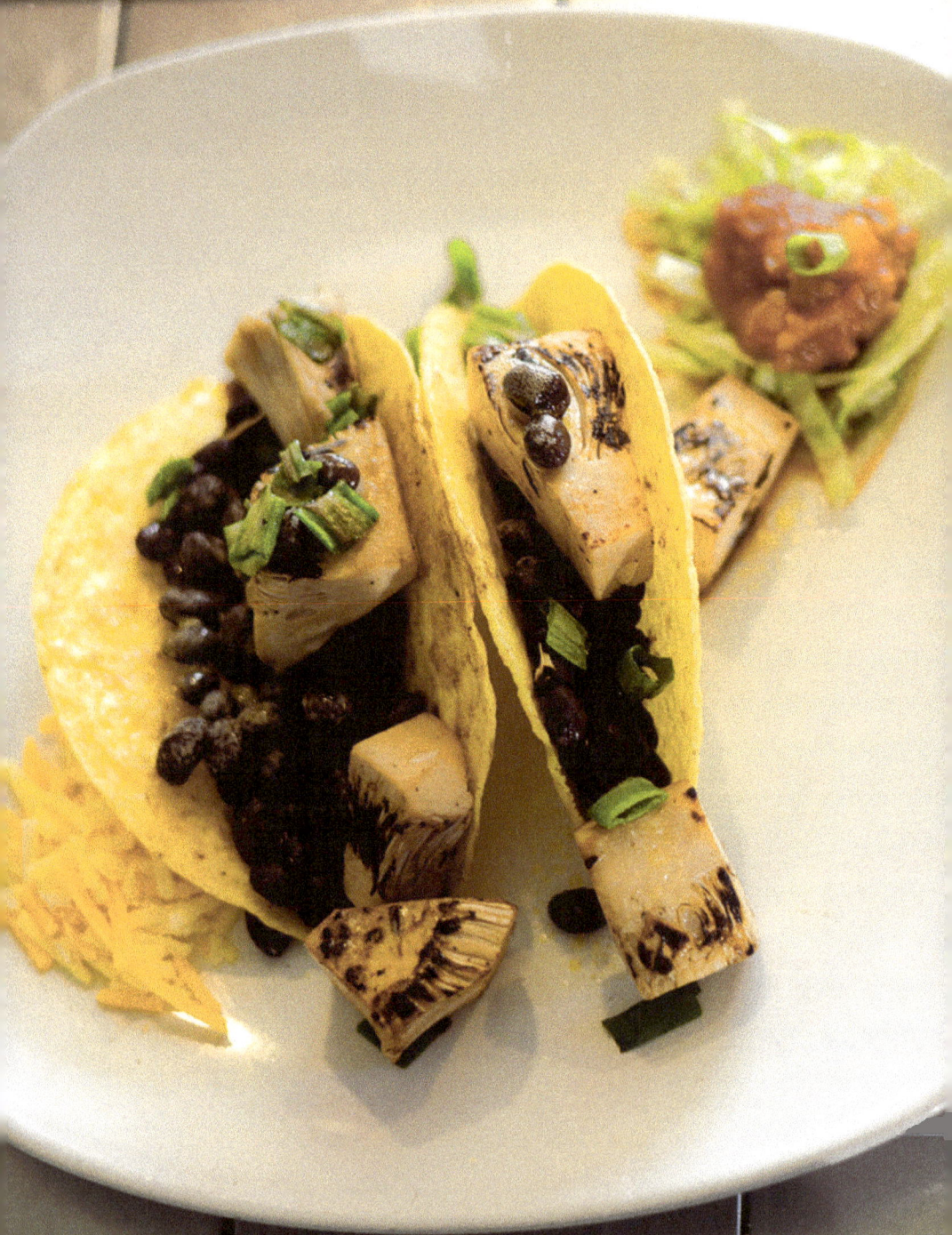

Jack-fruit & Black Bean Taco

Prepping Time: 15 minutes

Ingredients:

- 1 can of black beans
- 1 can of Jack fruit and drain liquid
- 1 Tablespoon of minced garlic
- ½ Teaspoon of cumin

- 1 ½ Cup of vegan cheese
- 1 ½ Cup of shredded lettuce
- 1 Diced tomato
- 2 Tablespoons of extra-virgin olive oil

- 4-6 Small taco shells hard or soft
- Cilantro & green onions

- Your favorite taco sauce

Directions:

- Sauté garlic in olive oil over medium heat in a small saucepan
- Add cumin and a pinch of salt while stirring for 30 seconds to 1 minute
- Add the canned beans & jack fruit and stir to combine
- Mash up the beans with a potato masher or fork
- Cook for just a few minutes but stir often until the mixture starts to simmer
- Reduce the heat & cover the pot. Stir every few minutes so the beans don't stick to the bottom of the pan
- Assemble your tacos: Spread a layer of beans down the center of each taco shell, followed by a small handful of lettuce, a drizzle of sauce and sprinkle of vegan cheese and cilantro and or green onions with diced tomato then serve immediately

Cooking Time: 15 minutes

Serves: 4-6 People

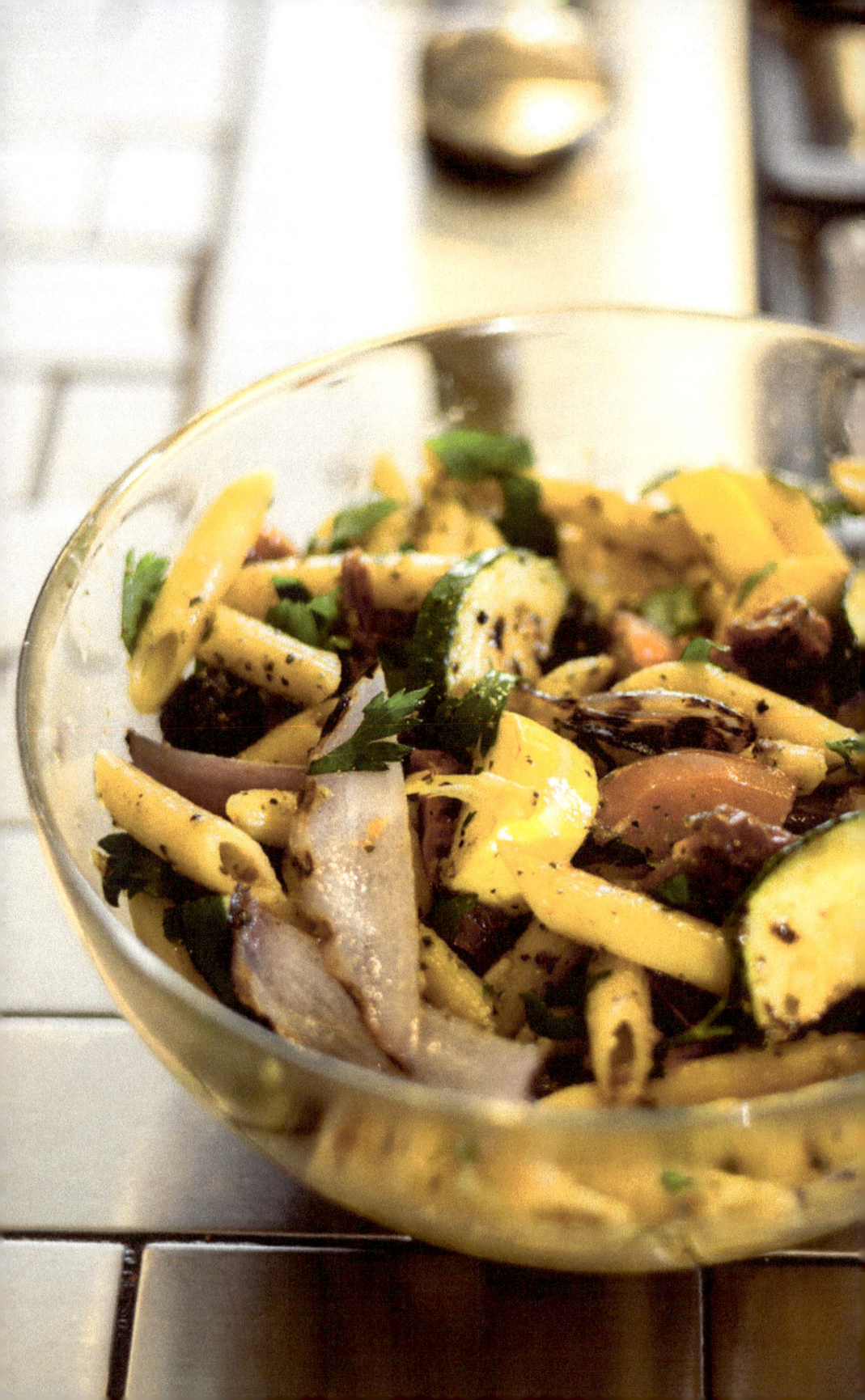

Mediterranean Vegetarian Pasta

Prepping Time: 15 minutes

Ingredients:

- 2 Plum tomatoes chopped
- Use Italian dressing or balsamic vinaigrette
- 6 Oz or (177 ml) cooked bowtie pasta
- ½ Zucchini & Squash sliced
- ¼ Red onion cut into chunks
- 2 Tablespoons of black olives sliced
- Add salt & pepper (for taste)

Directions:

- In a large bowl toss together vegetable ingredients with ¼ cup of vinaigrette/Italian dressing
- Let it marinate for 5 minutes while you preheat the grill
- Grill vegetables
- Add pasta, tomatoes, grilled vegetables, black olives & vinaigrette or Italian dressing to a bowl. Toss the ingredients together until coated and season with salt & pepper to desired taste

Cooking Time: 15 minutes

Serves: 4-6 People

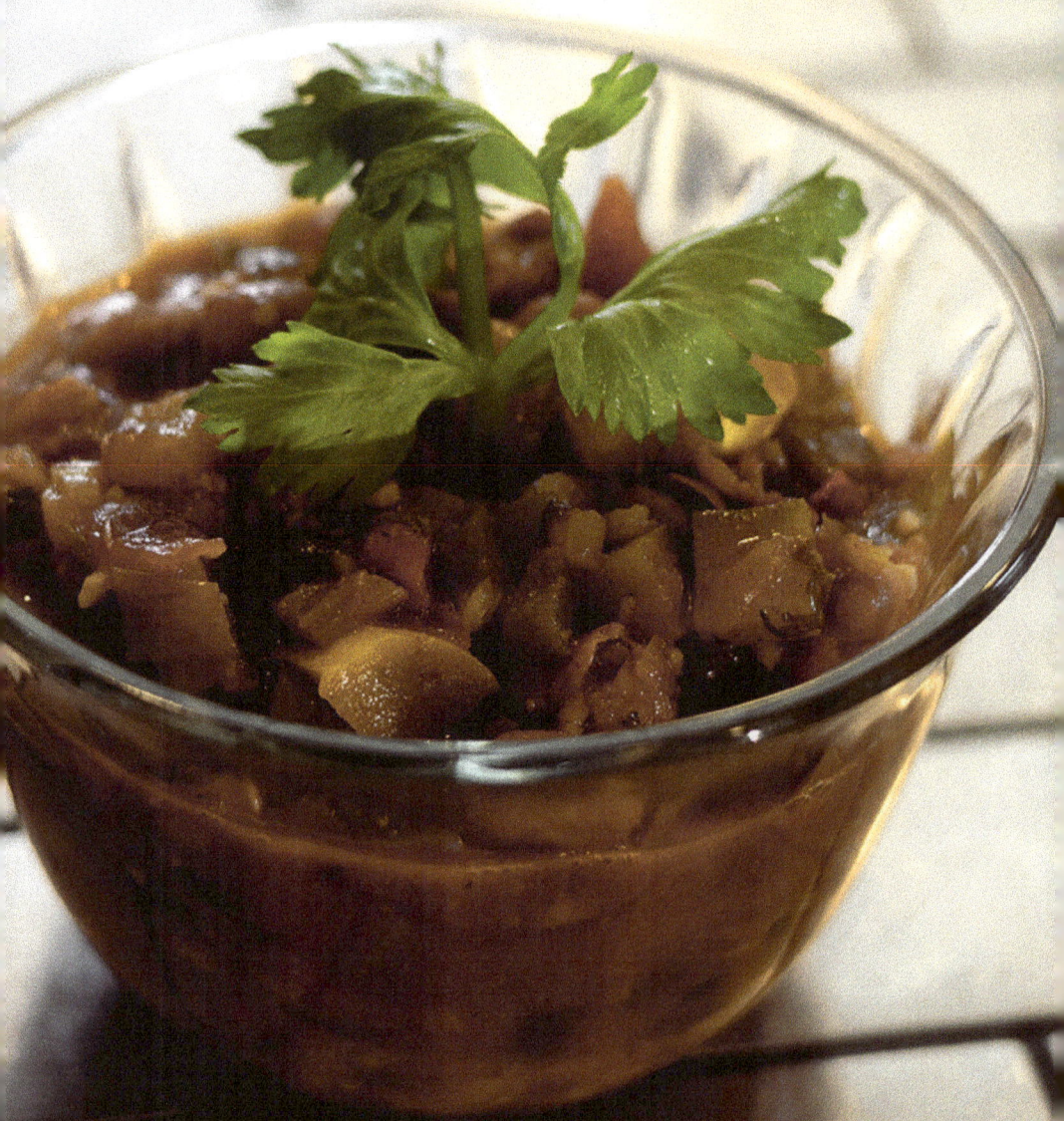

Vegetarian Chili

Prepping Time: 5 minutes

Ingredients:

- ½ Cup of chopped celery
- 1 Teaspoon of minced garlic
- 1 Cup of chopped onions
- 1 Cup of chopped red bell peppers (capsicum)
- 2 cans of tomatoes including the juice from the can

- 1 Cup of canned kidney beans rinsed and drained
- 1 Teaspoon of chili powder
- 1 Teaspoon of ground cumin
- 1 Teaspoon of Kosher salt

- 2 Tablespoons of Olive oil

Directions:

- Heat olive oil in a 10-inch pan over medium heat
- Add chopped onions, chopped celery and chopped red peppers (capsicum) and cook
- Stir occasionally for 2 minutes
- Stir in minced garlic, salt, cumin, chili powder and stir while cooking
- Add canned diced tomatoes, garbanzo and kidney beans and bring the mixture to a boil
- Once boiling reduce the heat to low and simmer for 15 minutes
- Place the chili into a bowl

Cooking Time: 15 minutes

Serves: 2 People

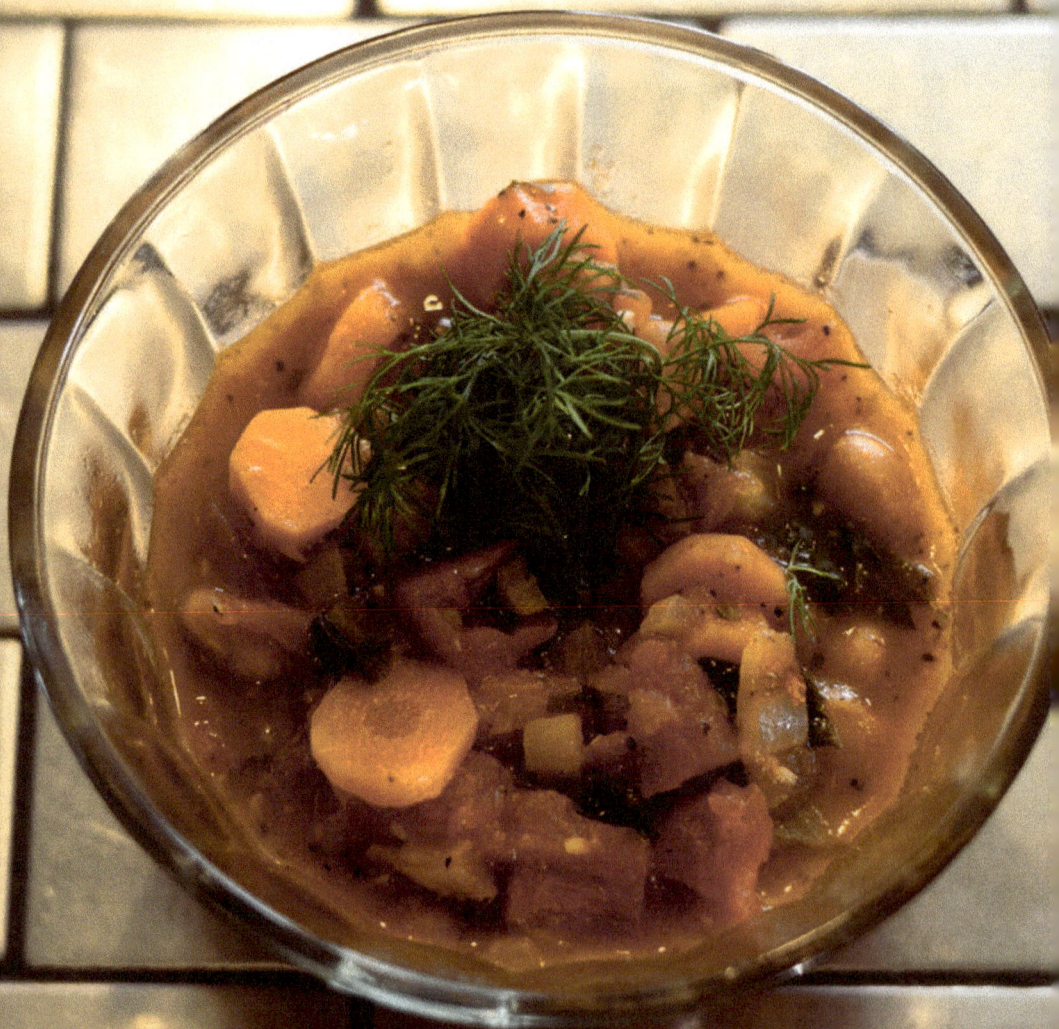

Vegetarian Minestrone Soup

Prepping Time: 5 minutes

Ingredients:

- ½ Teaspoon of dried basil, oregano, and thyme
- 1 Cup of chopped onions
- 2 Cloves of minced garlic
- 1 Celery rib diced
- 1 Carrot, peeled & diced
- 4 Cups of vegetable broth
- 1 can of diced tomatoes
- 1 Cup of pasta
- ½ Cup fresh or frozen green beans
- ½ Cup of canned red beans, rinsed 8 drained
- 2 Tablespoons of olive oil
- ½ Teaspoon salt
- ¼ Teaspoon of coarsely grounded black pepper

Directions:

- Heat olive oil in a pot
- Add onion, garlic, carrots and celery for about 5 minutes or until lightly browned
- Stir in vegetable broth, green beans, red beans, diced tomatoes, basil, oregano & thyme. Simmer on low for 20 minutes
- Add the pasta & cook until tender for about 10 minutes while stirring occasionally. You may add more broth if needed
- Season with salt & pepper
- Pour the soup into bowls and serve

Cooking Time: 30 minutes

Serves: 2 people

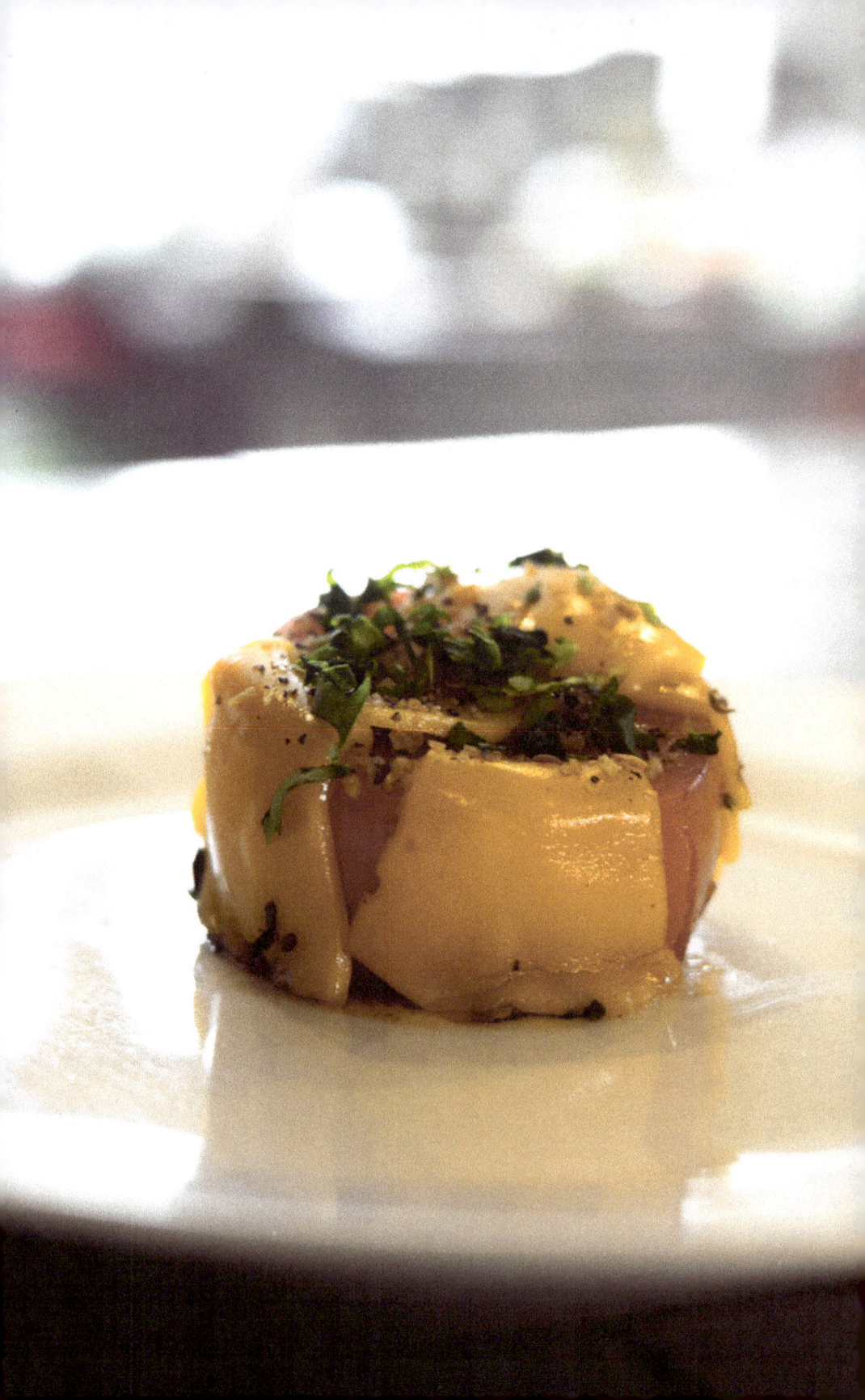

Vegetarian Tomato Bake

Prepping Time: 20 minutes

Ingredients:

- 2 Medium tomatoes
- 1 Teaspoon of olive oil
- Garlic powder
- Dried oregano
- Salt & pepper (for taste)

Directions:

- Preheat the over to 400 degrees (F) or (204 degrees Celsius)
- Line a baking sheet with parchment paper
- Add salt, garlic powder, oregano, and black pepper to a small bowl
- Slice a thin piece off the ends of each tomato
- Cut each tomato in half, in the middle
- Pat the tomatoes until dry and place them on the parchment paper lining-baking sheet. Arrange them so that they are not touching
- Bake the tomatoes for 5 minutes until the tomatoes soften
- Turn off the oven and turn on the broiler to low broil
- Broil the tomatoes for 1 ½ -2 minutes but keep an eye on them until lightly browned

Cooking Time: 12 minutes

Serves: 2 People

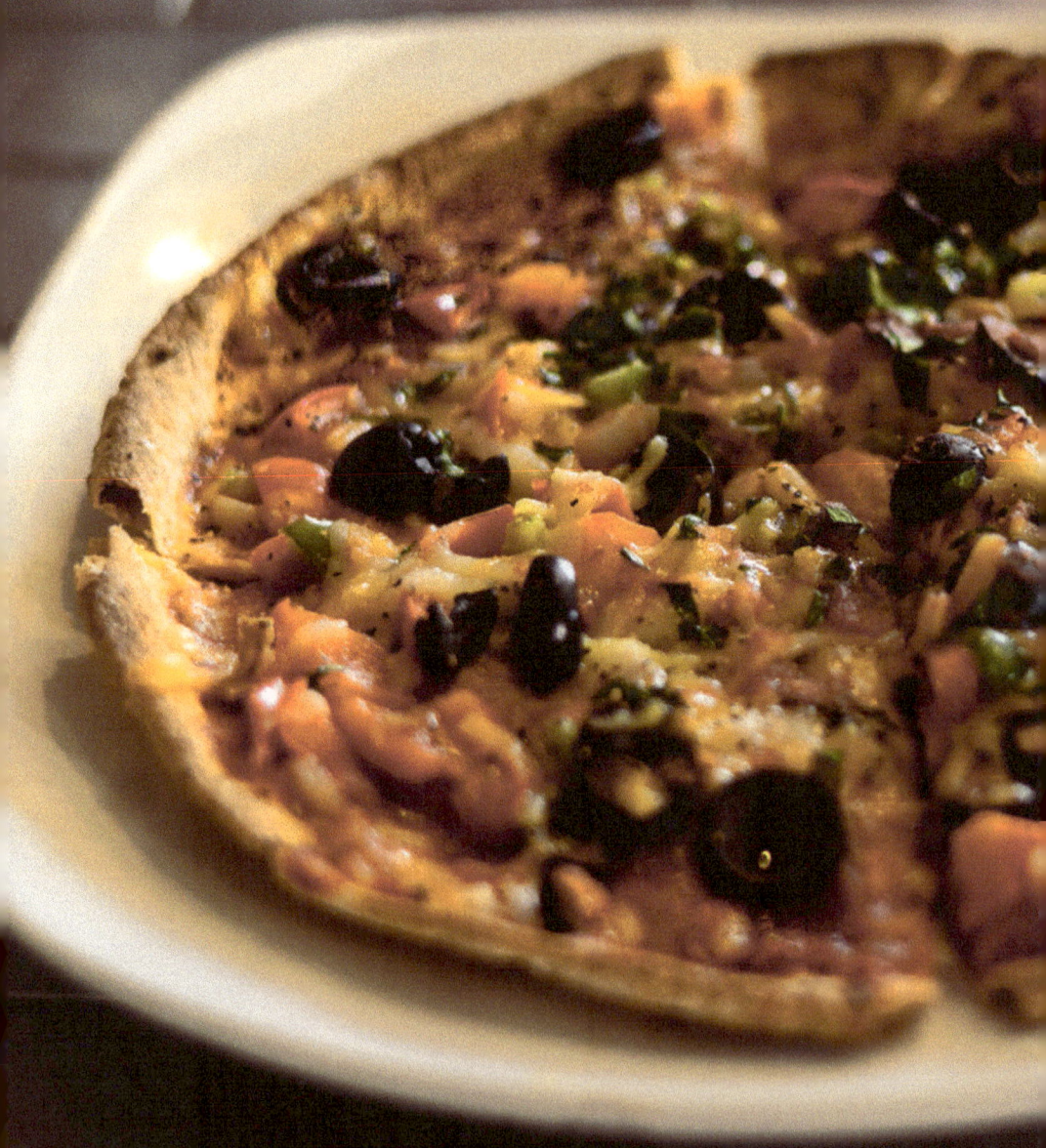

Vegetarian Flatbread Pizza

Prepping Time: 10 minutes

Ingredients:

- 10–12-inch thin crust pizza or flatbread
- Olive oil to sauté and to drizzle
- ¼ Cup of sliced red onions
- 1/3 Cup of red or green bell pepper (capsicum)
- ¼ Cup of tomatoes
- 1/3 Cup of olives
- ½ Cup (2 ounces) of cheese
- ½ Cup of torn basil or herbs of choice
- ½ Cup of tomato sauce

Directions:

- Preheat oven to 400 degrees (F) or (204 degrees Celsius) and line a baking sheet with parchment paper
- Place flat bread or pizza crust in the oven and lightly toast. Remove from oven and set aside
- Add tomato sauce and vegetables. Spread them all evenly on the flatbread or pizza crust
- Finish with cheese and herbs
- Place in oven on center rack until edges are crispy and the cheese is melted for about 10-15 minutes
- Remove and top with a dash of pepper, dash of sea salt and drizzle with olive oil

Cooking Time: 15 minutes

Serves: 3 People

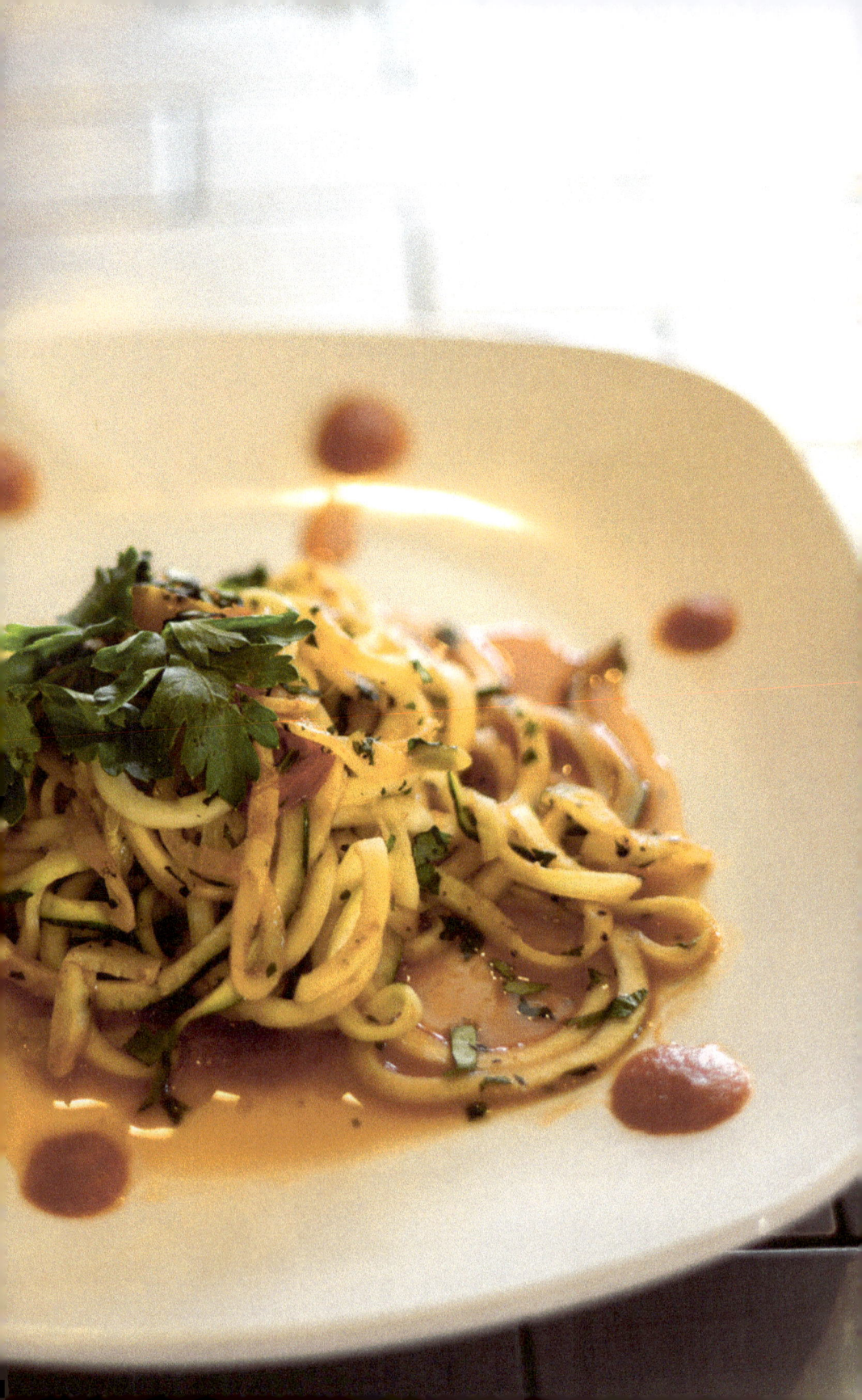

Vegetarian Zucchini Spaghetti

Prepping Time: 15 minutes

Ingredients:

- 2 Spiral cut zucchini
- 1 Tablespoon of minced garlic
- ¼ Cup of tomato sauce
- 1 Tablespoon of Parsley
- 1 Clove of minced garlic
- 1 Tablespoon of olive oil

Directions:

- Prepare zucchini noodles with spiral veggie cutter
- Sauté garlic & noodles in olive oil over medium heat until tender
- Add tomato sauce & toss until noodles are coated (add more sauce if needed)
- Sprinkle with salt & pepper (for desired taste)

Cooking Time: 15 minutes

Serves: 2 People

www.ingramcontent.com/pod-product-compliance
Lightning Source LLC
LaVergne TN
LVHW070013090426
835508LV00048B/3390